Plant-Based Diet for Weight Loss

The Paradox of an Introductory Guide on How to Kill Bad Habits so as not to Die of Fat (50 Delicious Bonus Recipes for the Vegetable-Based Diet)

By Michael Garavaglia

Table of Contents

Chapter 1: Introduction to Plant-Based Eating

The Importance of a Plant-based Diet for your Body and Health

The vegan diet or plant-based way of eating is a great way to improve your health and lifestyle by replacing all animal products and by-products with easy-to-digest plant-based foods. Following a plant-based diet has grown in popularity and is embraced by a lot of people, including celebrities, chefs, and ordinary people from all backgrounds. Some cultures embrace vegan meals and have for centuries, long before plant-based eating become more mainstream and available to everyone. There are many health benefits from switching to a vegan diet:

1. Weight loss is one of the major benefits of a plant-based diet. Many studies and research indicate that a diet without animal fats and protein is low in fat and contributes to lower rates of obesity, and on average, a healthier weight. This is due to the high fiber and low amount of fat in many fruits, vegetables, and other plant-based foods.

2. There is a high level of nutrients in a plant-based diet, as the foods include a wide variety of fruits and vegetables which contain numerous vitamins, minerals, antioxidants, and calcium. Certain vegetables contain a lot of protein, such as dark leafy greens kale, spinach, and arugula. Focusing on more varieties of plant-based foods can increase the number of nutrients in your diet.

3. Prevention of cancer is another benefit of a plant-based diet. Some research shows promising results on how changing to a vegan diet can prevent and reverse some forms of cancer. A high number of antioxidants, found in fresh fruits and vegetables, are responsible for slowing the formation of free radicals, which contribute to cancerous cell growth and other debilitating diseases and conditions. There is a lower rate of cancer among plant-based eaters, which is a good reason to ditch the meat.

4. Lower rates of heart disease and better blood pressure are benefits of a vegan diet, due to the lack of animal fats, which contribute to high blood pressure and clogged arteries, especially when consumed regularly. The elimination of meat increases heart health and helps prevent many chronic and more serious conditions that

can result from high blood pressure and related heart conditions.

5. Chronic conditions such as arthritis and fibromyalgia can be devastating for many people, though there are specific nutrients such as vitamin A and C can alleviate symptoms of these conditions and prevent inflammation and related pain that can result. Many fruits and vegetables contain anti-inflammatory properties that are beneficial for many conditions, by reducing pain and swelling.

6. Regulating insulin levels and maintaining healthy blood sugar levels are great benefits of the vegan diet. Fruits contain sugar, though the amount is enough for a healthy diet and is easily digested by the body, whereas refined and artificial forms of sugar contribute to high glucose levels, which increase the risk of Type 2 Diabetes.

7. Plant-based eaters often report higher levels of energy, which makes it easier to stay active, exercise and keep weight at a reasonable level.

8. A vegan diet can improve the health of skin, nails, and hair by reducing the number of blemishes and breakouts.

9. In some cases, vegan diets can be less expensive and easier to shop for than diets that include meat, fish, and dairy products, which are often costly. Beans, grains, legumes, nuts, and seeds, all of which are plant-based and full of nutrients, can be purchased in bulk and enjoyed in small amounts as an important part of your eating plan.

10. Plant-based eating can help alleviate many other conditions, including high cholesterol, digestive conditions, and nutrient deficiencies. Due to contrary belief, a vegan diet can meet all your nutrient requirements, including B12 and vitamin D.

Exploring new foods and recipes is an excellent way to adapt to a plant-based diet, which doesn't need to occur overnight. It's best to gradually introduce new foods into the diet and discover which ones you like the best for future menu and meal planning. Often, people focus on dietary restrictions, instead of enjoying the amount of flexibility and new opportunities many foods provide. A plant-based diet is a scientifically proven healthy way to eat and enjoy food for a lifetime, and you'll love the benefits it provides!

The Impact of Eating Processed Foods and Meat on Weight Gain and Disease

Many people enjoy a wider variety of foods on a vegan diet. This is not just because they are simply replacing meat and dairy products, but rather, focusing on the wide range of foods that are plant-based. Over time, you'll notice some major improvements to your health and well-being, which includes losing excess weight and improving your metabolism. Meat products may seem like a good choice in dieting, especially when choosing lean meats and fish. However, there are a lot of pesticides and chemicals used in processing meats that can impact our bodies and how we digest them. There are also growing concerns about the treatment of animals in factory farming and how this impacts their lives as well as ours. Choosing vegan not only makes a healthier lifestyle but a more ethical one as well.

Chapter 2: How to Start a New Diet Plan and Ditch Unhealthy Habits

Focus on Plant-Based Proteins and Nutrients

Choosing the right plant-based protein for your diet is easier than you think, and there are more options than most people realize. Many of the common vegetable proteins on the market tend to be more versatile and available in a variety of forms and textures, which makes adding them to your diet effortless. In fact, there is a much wider range of plant-based protein than animal-based.

Soy Products

One of the most popular and commonly purchased vegan proteins is soy. Tofu, tempeh, miso, soymilk, and other dairy-free products are included in this category. Tempeh and miso are fermented forms of soy and contain B12, calcium, protein, and fiber. They are excellent additions to any meal, including soups, stir fry dishes, roasts, and salads. Tofu remains a common option for vegans and contains a high amount of both protein and calcium. Soy-based drinks and dairy replacements are often soy-based, such as yogurts, creams, cheese, and milk.

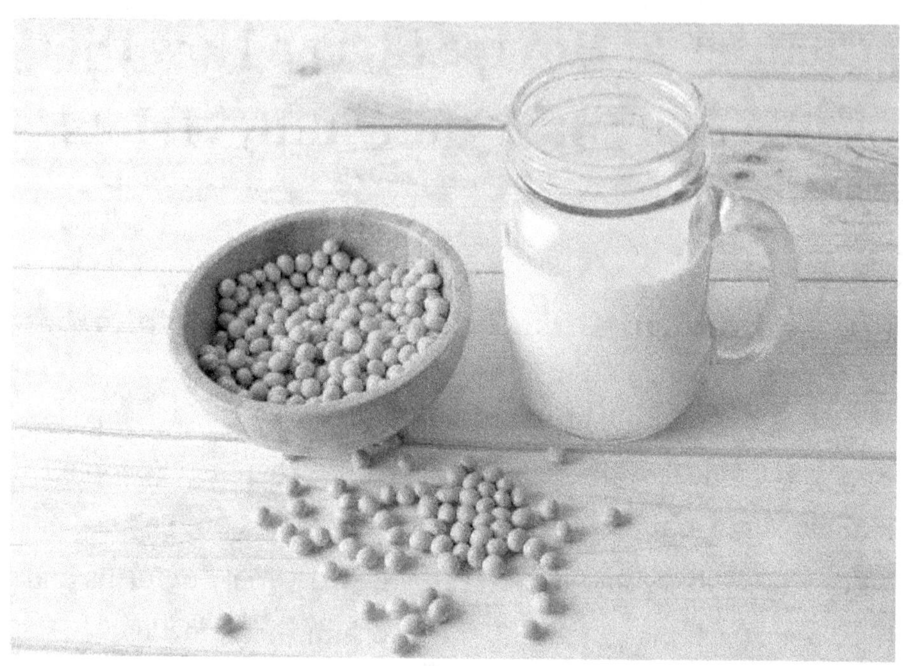

Seitan

This protein source is made from gluten, which is found in whole wheat. It is a form of protein that is made by isolating the gluten or protein content from the wheat. This process of making seitan is usually time-consuming, and not often the most commonly used vegan protein, though it is a good option for people with soy allergies. Seitan should be avoided by people who are gluten intolerant. It can be found in some natural food stores.

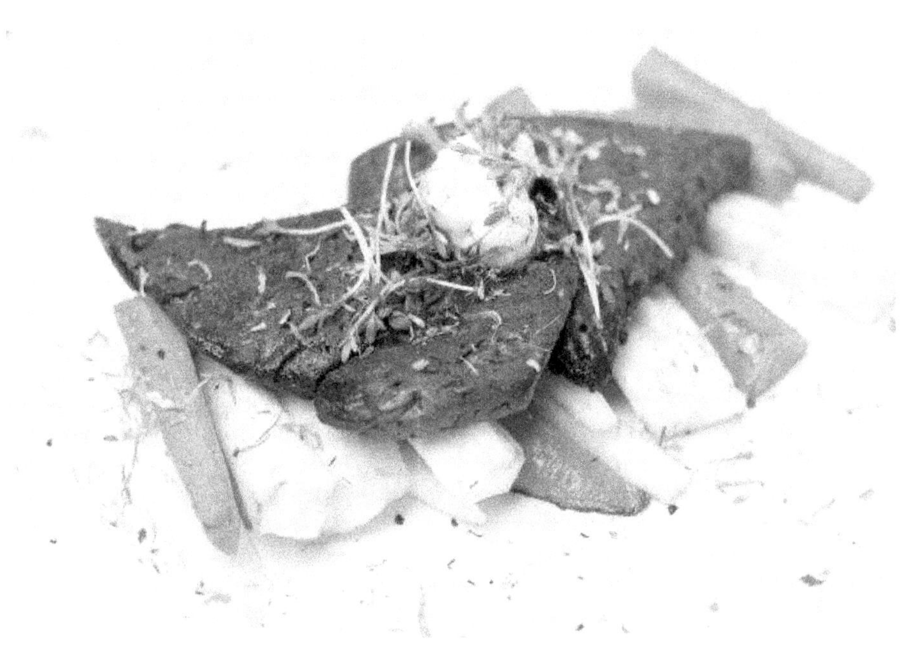

Lentils

These beans are easy to cook and don't require the soaking time that kidney beans, chickpeas, black beans, and other varieties require. They are flavorful and can be easily added to soups, stews, and salads. On their own, they can create tasty dishes full of spice.

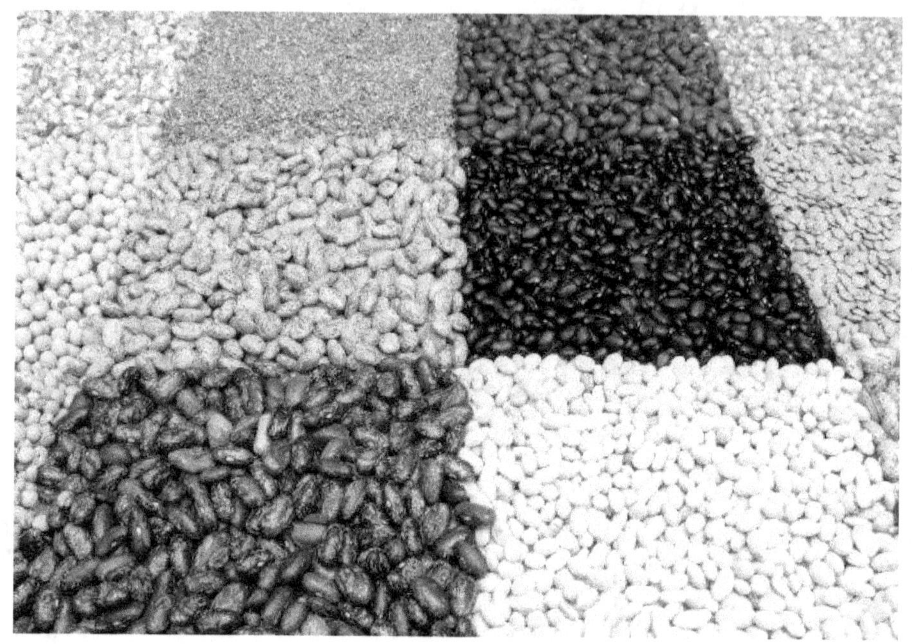

Chickpeas

A good source of protein and fiber, chickpeas are always good to have in the pantry for many soups, salads, and stews. Canned or dried, chickpeas are inexpensive and easy to add to a variety of meals

Quinoa

It's often considered both a grain and a pulse. Quinoa is a high-protein food with amino acids that can take the place of rice and other sides in many dishes. It's a great side dish on its own, or as a supplement to stews and soups. Many salads add quinoa to boost the fiber and protein content.

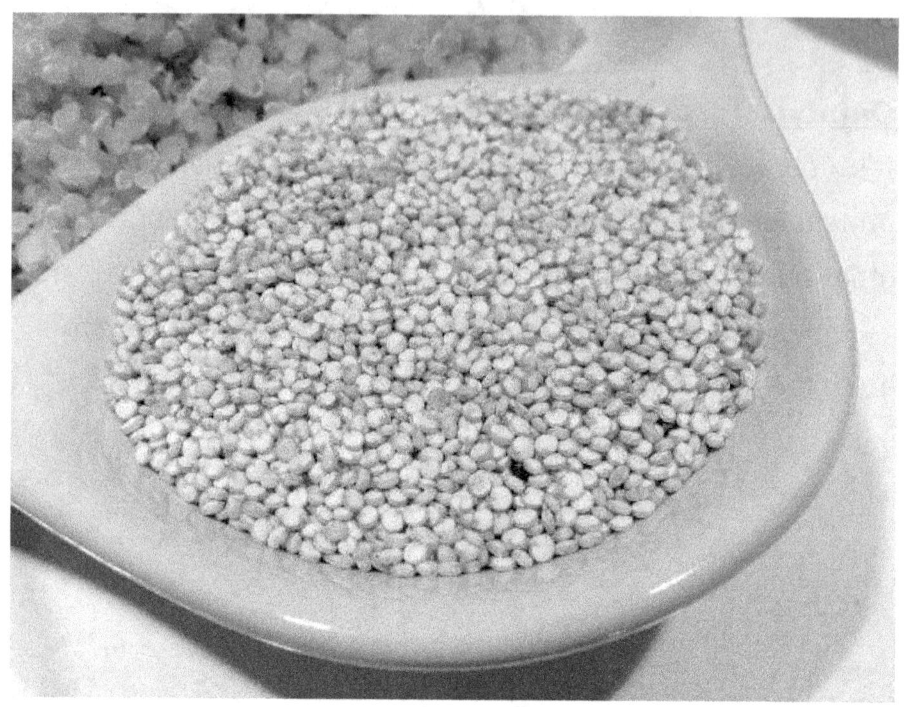

Green Peas

A sweet, flavorful vegetable, green peas are a good protein source. They are also high in fiber and make a pleasant ingredient in soups and baked dishes, such as shepherd's pie and other casseroles.

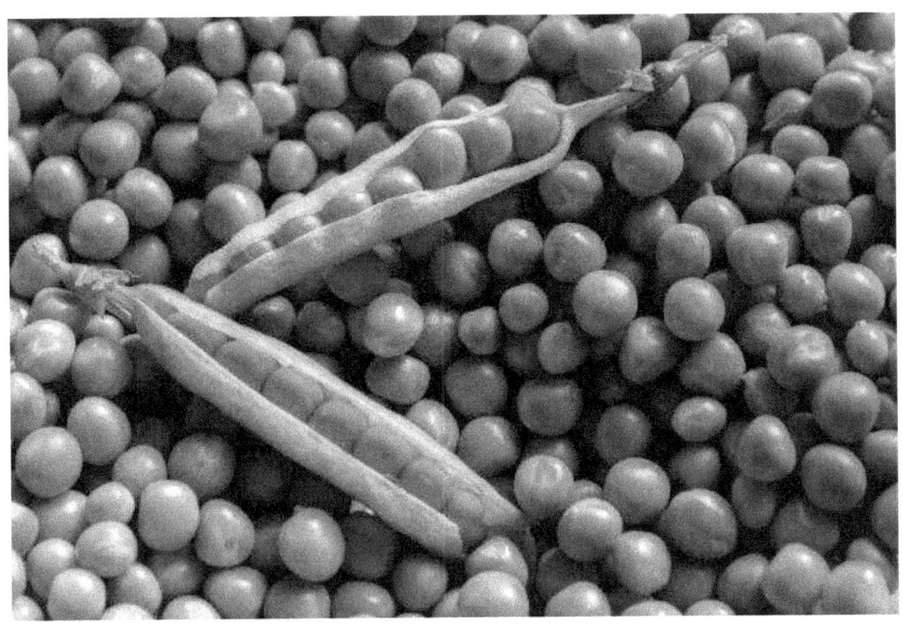

Foods to Choose for Your Diet: Keeping it Healthy and Vegan

Creating a shopping list can be a challenging experience when there are changes to your diet or the need to work within budgetary constraints. When choosing plant-based foods, concentrate on the fresh produce and natural foods as much as possible, avoiding packaged and artificially flavored options. This is especially important for ensuring you get the most nutrients possible while having access to a variety of choices. The following selection of items provides a good start for building your shopping list.

Fresh (and Frozen) Produce Section

This section of the grocery store is located around the perimeters of the store and contains the bulk of items you'll need for your shopping trip. Most stores contain a good variety of options, and wherever possible, it's best to choose fruits and vegetables in season, as they are fresh and locally harvested. If there are specific fruits or vegetables unavailable in the produce section, they may be found in the frozen section. Frozen is the next best option after fresh, and if neither is an option, choose canned.

Dark leafy greens are one of the most highly nutritious vegetables you can include in your diet, and are especially important for vegans, due to the high calcium and fiber content. Kale, arugula, and spinach are among the most nutrient-rich in the dark greens. For vegetables high in vitamin C, choose bell peppers. Onions and garlic are also useful for flavoring a wide variety of meals, as well as dried or fresh herbs and spices. Cabbage, green peas, carrots, squash, potatoes, and yams are among some of the best vegetables for creating a lot of meals, and they tend to be inexpensive and readily available in most stores.

Citrus fruits are a good source of vitamin C, while berries are high in antioxidants in general. Apples and bananas make excellent snacks on their own, because of their portability: they are already "packaged" in their skin and can be taken on the go for convenient snacking anywhere. Pomegranates and avocados are especially rich in vitamins and should be considered when they are available, even if you only purchase one or two.

Soy Products and Dairy Alternatives

During your shopping trip, you'll notice the tofu, sprouts, and many meat-free and dairy alternatives are located close to (or right in) the produce section. This is a convenient location for combining your vegetable proteins with your grocery selection. Tofu is usually available in a variety of flavors, alongside tempeh and an array of dairy-free cheeses, "meat" balls, patties, and sausages. Miso paste is usually available in this area, or where other soups can be found.

Sprouts, herbs, and spices

These can be purchased dry or fresh. If you choose fresh, make sure they are used quickly to avoid wilting. Sprouts must also be used within a day or so in order to keep the freshness and quality of nutrients available. Some stores offer these products in bulk, which can be helpful if you only require a small portion at a time.

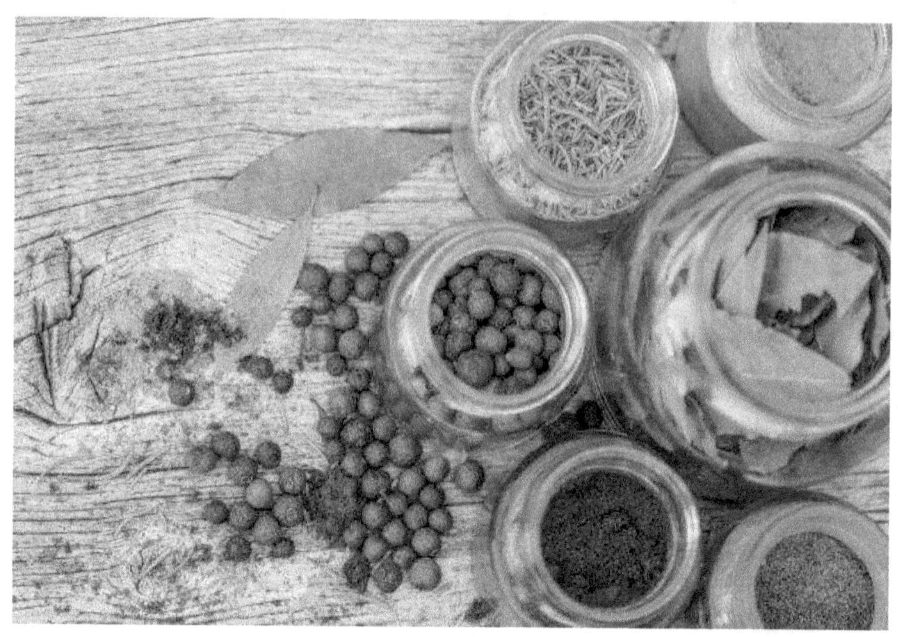

Nuts and Seeds

Pumpkin, sesame, chia, flax, and hemp seeds are all high in protein, fatty acids, and vitamins. Chia seeds are the most nutrient-dense of these seeds and can be found in natural food stores, as well as many regular grocery stores. Nuts are a good snack and topping or addition to many dishes. These can be found in the bulk aisle or close to the snack section. Most people skip these foods, not realizing their potential.

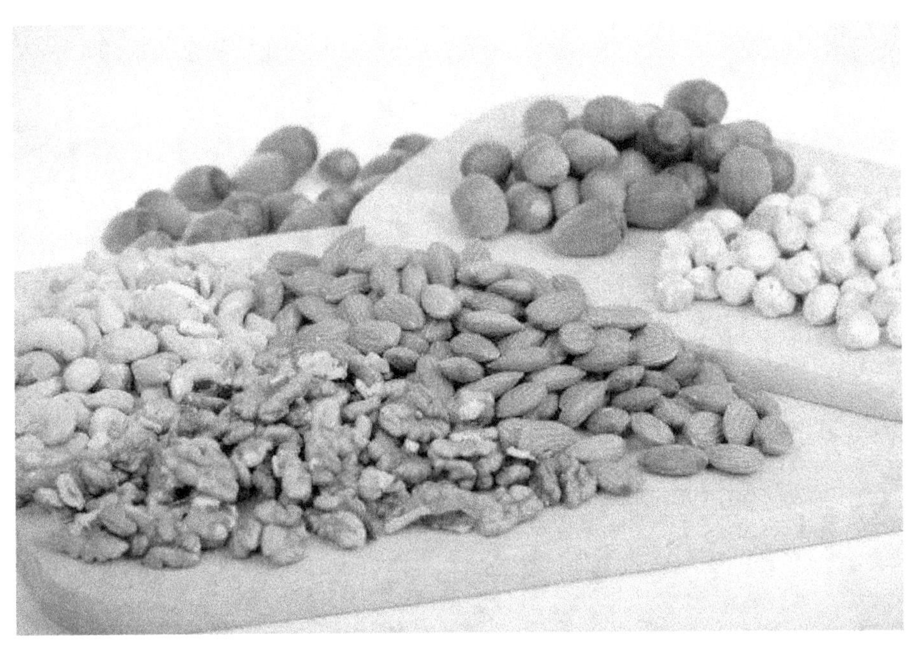

Diary-Free Milk and Vegan Alternatives to Dairy Products

Soymilk is the most common and frequently used non-dairy beverage, though there are a growing number of other options, including coconut, hazelnut, rice, and almond milk. Hemp and oats milk are also options in some natural food stores. Dairy-free yogurt, cheese, sour cream, and butter are often found in the dairy section and/or with the assortment of tofu and other plant-based options in the produce section.

Shopping for a plant-based diet means avoiding some key areas around the grocery store or market, as well as many foods that are not suitable or healthy. Some vegan foods can be unhealthy if they contain a lot of preservatives or artificial ingredients, such as some packaged vegan "meats" and cheeses. It's best to use your own discretion to determine which options work best for you.

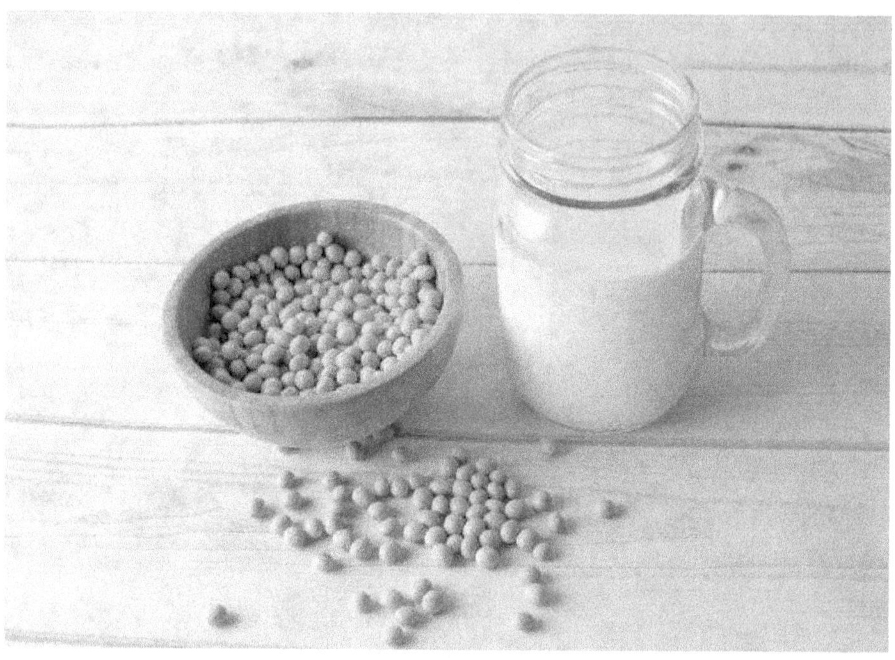

Foods to Avoid on a Vegan Diet

The following foods are best to avoid on a vegan diet, whether they are animal-based, meat by-products, or simply not a good choice for optimal health and weight loss:

- Flavored, processed vegan "meats", such as faux sausages, burgers, and cheeses with a lot of artificial ingredients. Some are better options than others, which can be researched and determined ahead of your next shopping trip

- Meat and dairy products. With the exception of some soy-based and dairy-free milk and related items located in the dairy section, all other foods should be skipped, including meats, dairy, and eggs.

- Sugary and high sodium snacks are best to avoid, as they can be easily replaced with nuts, seeds, and fresh fruits.

- Soda and fruit juice are high in sugar and will work against your efforts to lose weight and keep it off. For this reason, avoid these drinks altogether, and choose sparkling water (with natural flavor), coffee, tea, and water.

- Ice cream is another option that should be avoided, although there are some vegan options that can serve as a treat on occasion.

- Baked goods, bread, and cakes should generally be avoided unless you are aware of dairy-free bread or baked foods are options. Pastries and other sweet bakery treats are best to avoid because of their high sugar content. Some bakeries feature vegan baking, which can be a nice indulgence on occasion.

Make a list of grocery items and/or categories of the foods you want to include in your next shopping trip to make the task much easier. You'll find that shopping vegan is much easier, as you will only need to focus your attention on certain areas of the store. It may seem to limit at first, however, once you observe the full range of foods and options within these categories, you may be tempted to try new foods and flavors you may never have considered before, making your shopping experience more of an adventure.

Chapter 3: 10 Easy Smoothies for Breakfast

Breakfast Smoothies for a quick breakfast on the go. They provide a good portion of nutrients, many of which meet our body's daily requirements. There are many options for plant-based smoothies, including a wide range of fruits, non-dairy milk options, sweeteners, and spices. The best options for sweeteners are maple syrup and low carb options, such as swerve and monk fruit.

Avocado Banana Smoothie

This is a nutrient-rich smoothie that works to give you an abundance of energy and fiber in one serving. The combination of bananas and avocado provides a good serving of protein, healthy fats, potassium, and antioxidants. The milk used in this recipe is coconut due to its thick consistency, which creates a creamy texture, though almond and other nut milk are good choices as well.

- 1 ripe avocado
- 1 banana

- 2 cups of coconut milk (or another dairy-free option)

- 2 tablespoons of natural sweetener

- ½ cups of ice

Blend the milk, avocado, and banana together, then add in the sweetener and pulse briefly. Ice can be added and crushed to chill before serving. Makes two servings. The preparation time is five minutes.

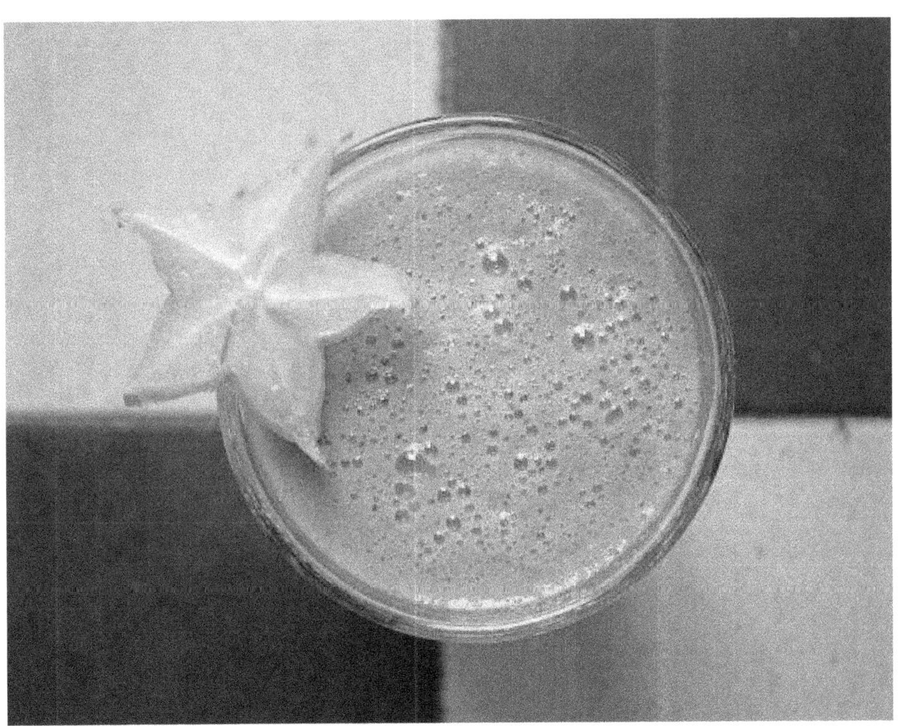

Coconut Yogurt Berry Smoothie

A dairy-free yogurt is an option if you're interested in trying coconut cultured yogurt, which contains many of the same nutrients and probiotics as the dairy version, only without any animal byproducts. This type of vegan yogurt is popular in some natural food stores and is becoming increasingly more available in regular grocery stores. The best option for smoothies is plain or vanilla, though if you want to reduce the level of sugar in your diet, then plain and unsweetened is the best option.

- 1 cup of coconut yogurt

- 1 cup of fresh or frozen berries

- ½ of a banana

- 1 teaspoon vanilla extract

- 2 cups of coconut or almond milk

- 1 tablespoon sweetener

Combine and blend the coconut yogurt and milk for 30 seconds, then add the berries, banana, vanilla extract, and sweetener, and pulse for one minute. If desired, add some ice to crush into the smoothie, then serve.

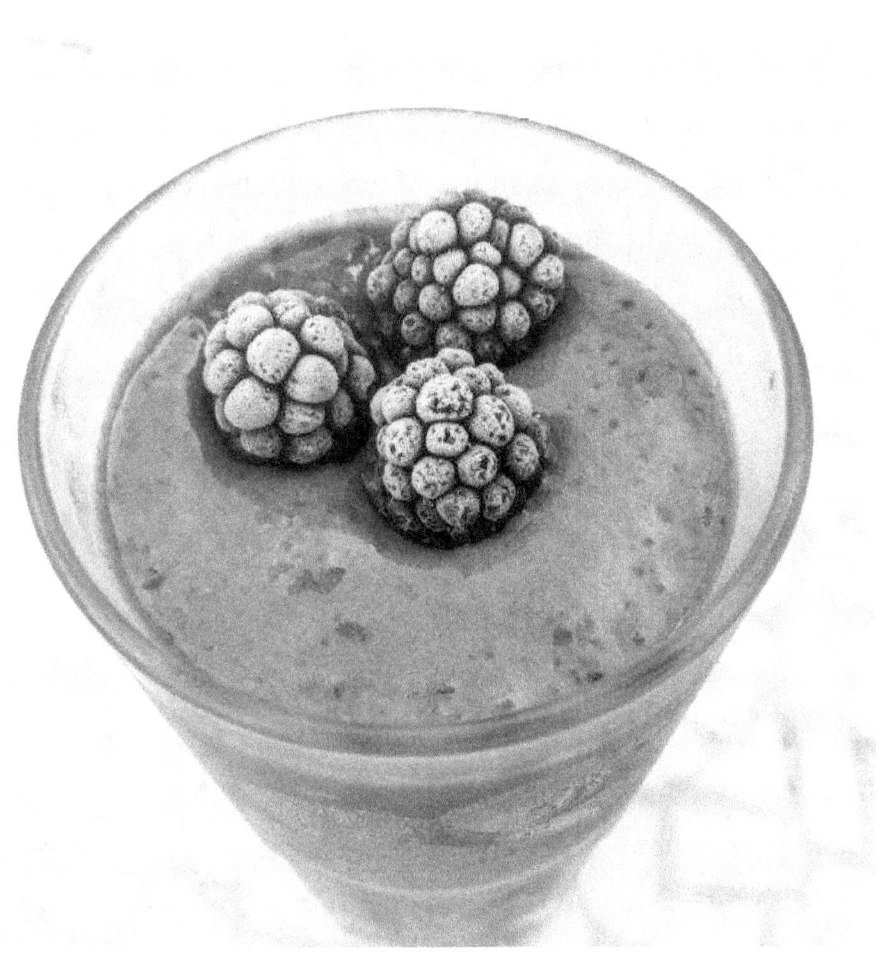

Almond Cocoa Energy Smoothie

Almonds are an excellent source of protein. This recipe blends cocoa powder, almond milk, and almond butter to create a thick, delicious treat that satisfies your hunger and nutrient needs. This smoothie is a great option for protein and energy just before the gym.

- 2 tablespoons cocoa powder

- 2 tablespoons natural sweetener

- 2 cups of almond milk

- ½ cups of almond butter

Blend almond milk and butter together for 30 seconds, then add in the sweetener and cocoa powder and pulse for another 30 seconds or until smooth. Makes two servings. Preparation time: five minutes.

There are a few variations to consider for this recipe:

- Add a banana for a thicker smoothie

- 1 teaspoon of the almond extract can be added to strengthen the almond flavor.

- Replace the almond butter with another nut-based butter, such as peanut butter, tahini, or hazelnut butter

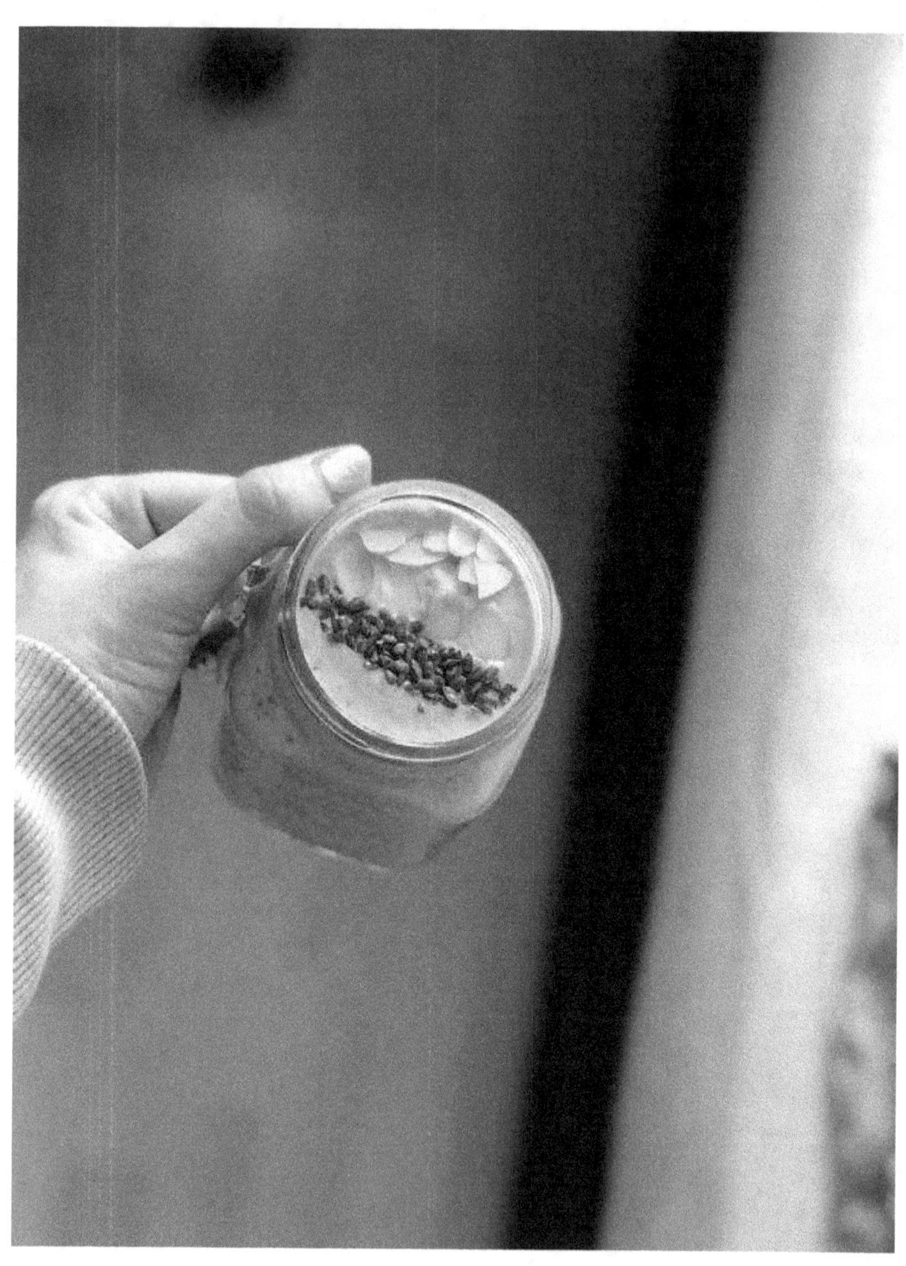

Pumpkin Cinnamon Smoothie

This smoothie is a variation on a pumpkin spice theme, by minimizing the number of spices to just cinnamon to keep it simple. If desired, pumpkin spice or the combination of cinnamon, nutmeg, and cloves can also be added for a full pumpkin spice flavor.

- ½ of a banana

- 2 teaspoons of cinnamon

- 2 teaspoons natural sweetener

- 1 cup of pumpkin puree (canned or fresh, with seeds removed)

- 2 cups of almond milk

The pumpkin puree and almond milk should be blended first in a blender until they are smoothly combined. Add the banana, sweetener, and cinnamon and process for another 30 seconds. Serves two portions and preparation time is two to five minutes.

Do you want to make this a pumpkin spice smoothie? Replace the cinnamon in this recipe with the following:

- ¼ teaspoon of cloves

- 1 teaspoon of nutmeg

- 1 teaspoon of cinnamon

Combine the three spices in a small, separate bowl, and blend with the ingredients. The banana can be substituted with an extra ½ cup of pumpkin puree.

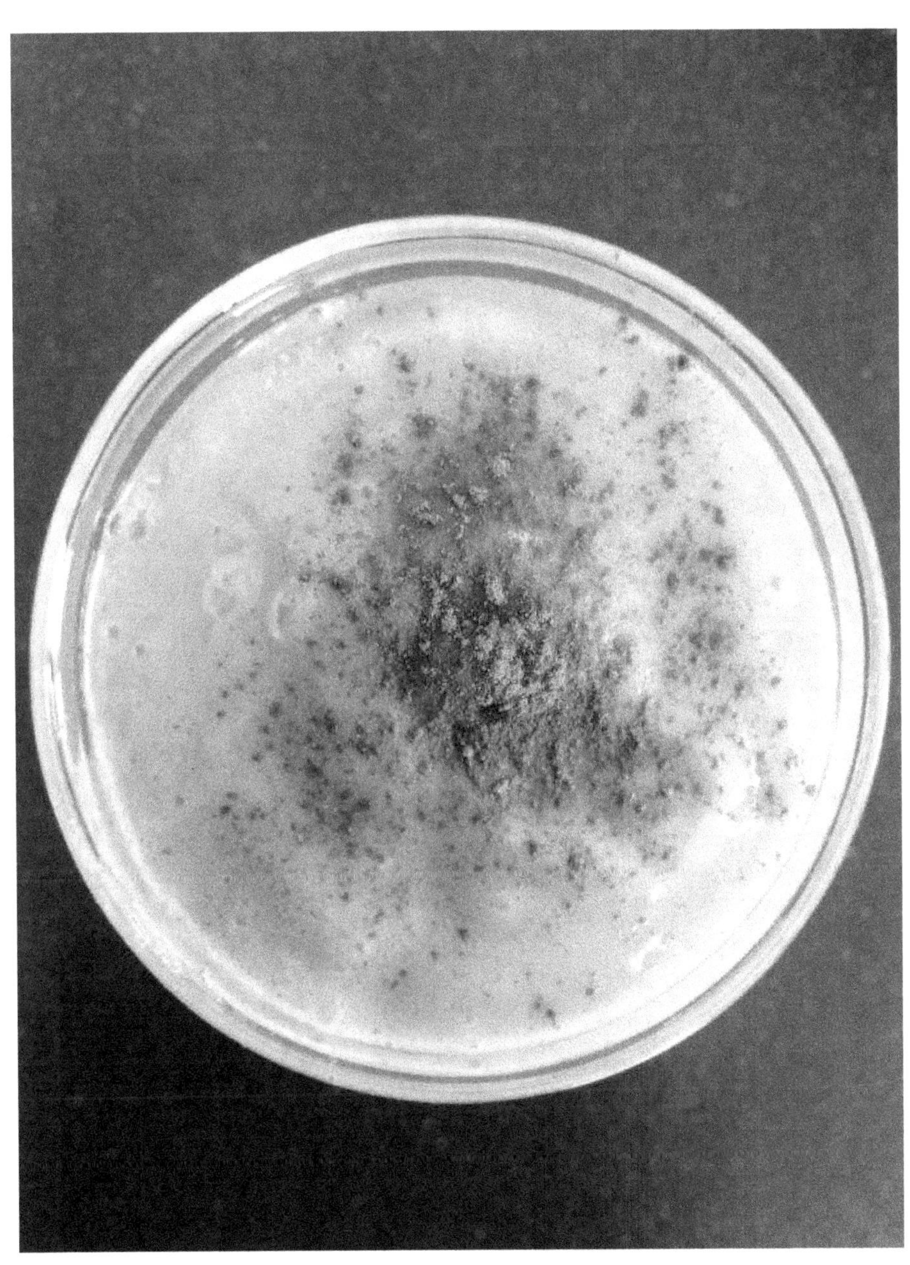

Cherries and Peaches Smoothie

Cherries are naturally sweet to taste, and a scoop of sweetener may not be needed in this smoothie. Coupled with a fresh peach, this recipe is an ideal treat at any time of the day, including breakfast. Cherries are high in alkaline, which helps with digestion and reducing pain from inflammation.

- I large ripe peach (soft), pit removed and sliced

- 1 cup of put cherries (fresh or frozen)

- 2 cups of coconut or almond milk

- 1 tablespoon of natural sweetener (optional)

- 1 teaspoon of vanilla extract (optional)

- ½ cups of crushed ice

Combine and mix the milk and cherries for 20 seconds, then add in the peach, sweetener, and vanilla, and blend again, then add in the ice. This smoothie serves two and takes five minutes to prepare.

Variations on the recipe include the following:

- Replace the peach with a ripe mango

- Instead of cherries, use 1 cup of raspberries

- Add a banana to thicken the drink

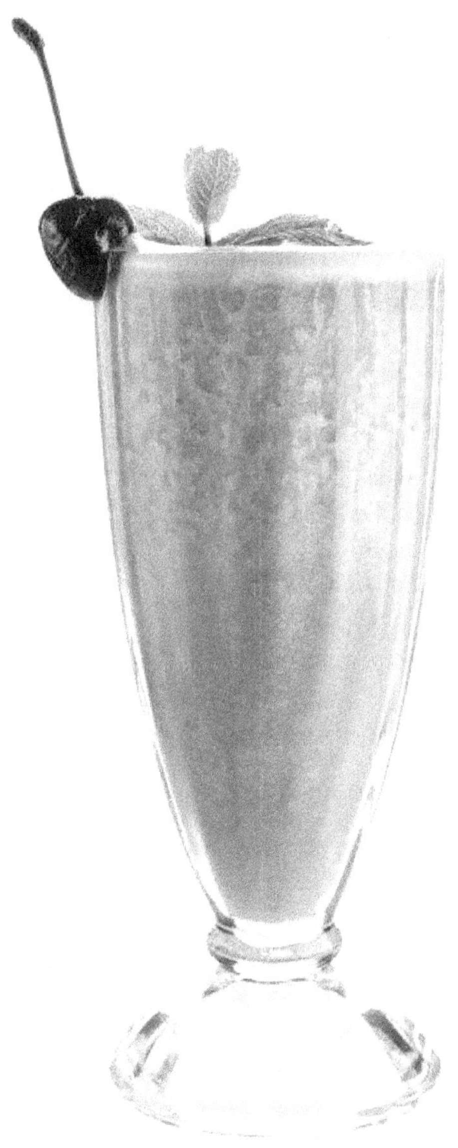

Mango Pistachio Smoothie

Mangoes are sweet and make an excellent ingredient for smoothies for this reason. Their flavor works well with a variety of other fruits, such as pineapple, coconut, papaya, and banana. Pistachios are added to boost this smoothie with a dose of protein.

- ¼ cups if crushed pistachios

- 2 cups of coconut milk

- ½ cups of coconut yogurt

- 2 medium mangoes, pits removed and sliced

- 2 teaspoons of natural sweetener

- ½ of a banana (optional)

Blend the milk, yogurt, and mangoes together and blend for 20 seconds. Add in the sweetener, banana (optional) and pistachios and continue to mix. If needed, add more milk if the smoothie becomes too thick. Top with pistachios before serving. This recipe makes two servings and the preparation time is five minutes.

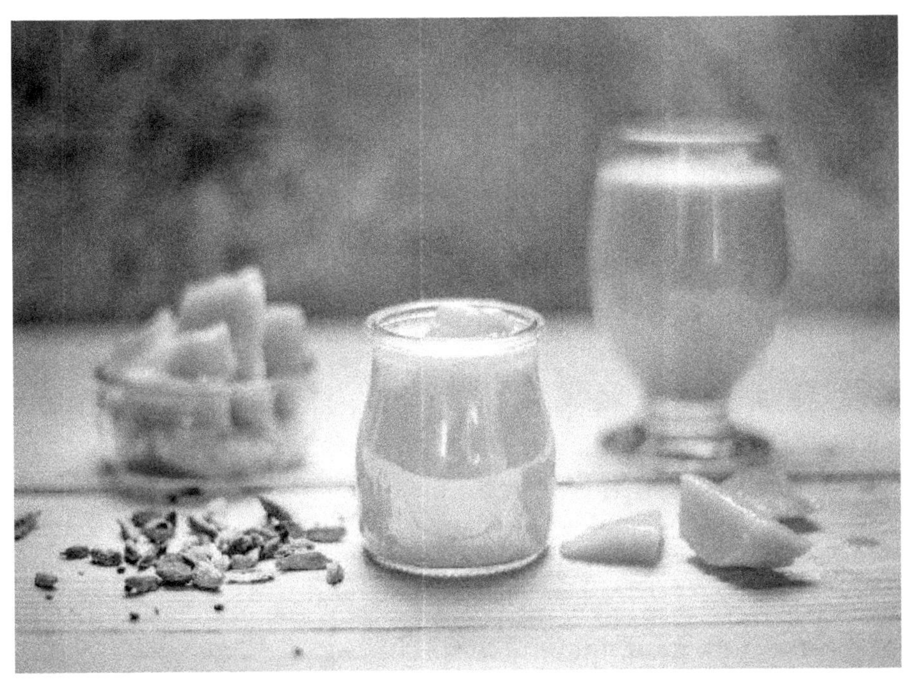

Kiwi, Strawberry, and Banana Smoothie

The sweetness of strawberries combined with the sour taste of kiwis creates a tasty blend with a banana and milk. Blackberries, raspberries, or blueberries can be added or used in place of the strawberries when they are not available.

- 1 cup of strawberries (sliced and stems removed)

- 1 kiwi, sliced and peeled

- 2 tablespoons of sweetener

- 2 cups of almond milk

- 1 banana

Combine the milk, banana, and berries in the blender and mix. Then, add in the kiwi and sweetener and blend for another 20 seconds, until smooth, then serve. This recipe makes two servings and takes 6-8 minutes to prepare.

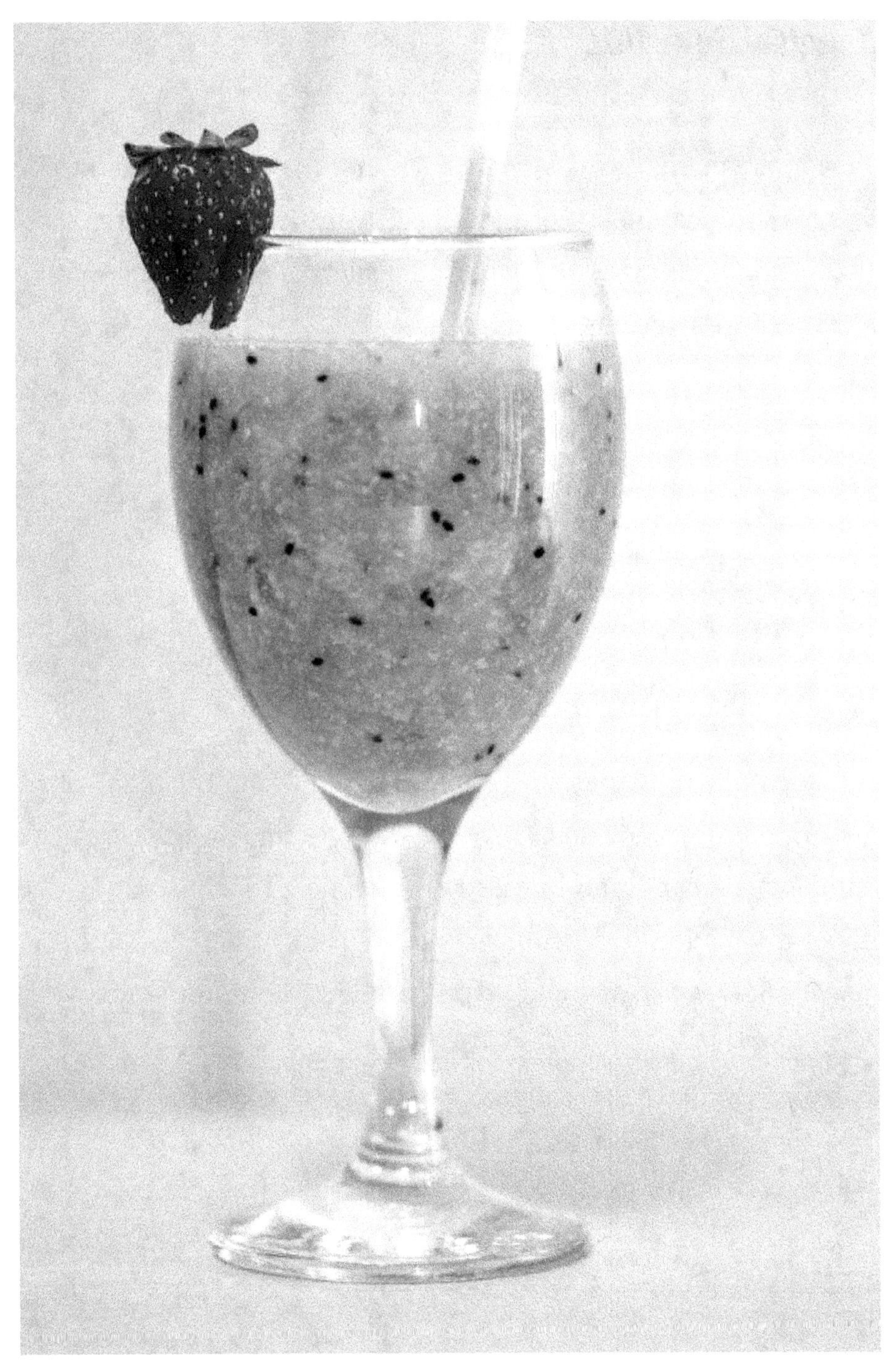

Tropical Smoothie

Pineapple, mango, papaya, and coconut milk are combined to create a tropical-inspired smoothie. This is a tasty, rich treat that can include other tropical fruits, such as guava and banana, or other fruits available to use.

- 1 cup of pineapple, sliced

- 1 cup of papaya, sliced

- ½ cups of sliced mangoes

- 2 cups of coconut milk

- 2 tablespoons of sweetener

Add the milk, mangoes, pineapple, and papaya to the blender and pulse for 30 seconds, then add the sweetener and pulse for another 10 seconds, adding extra milk if needed (this may be necessary if additional fruits are added, such as bananas and/or guava). Serves two and can be prepared in 6-8 minutes.

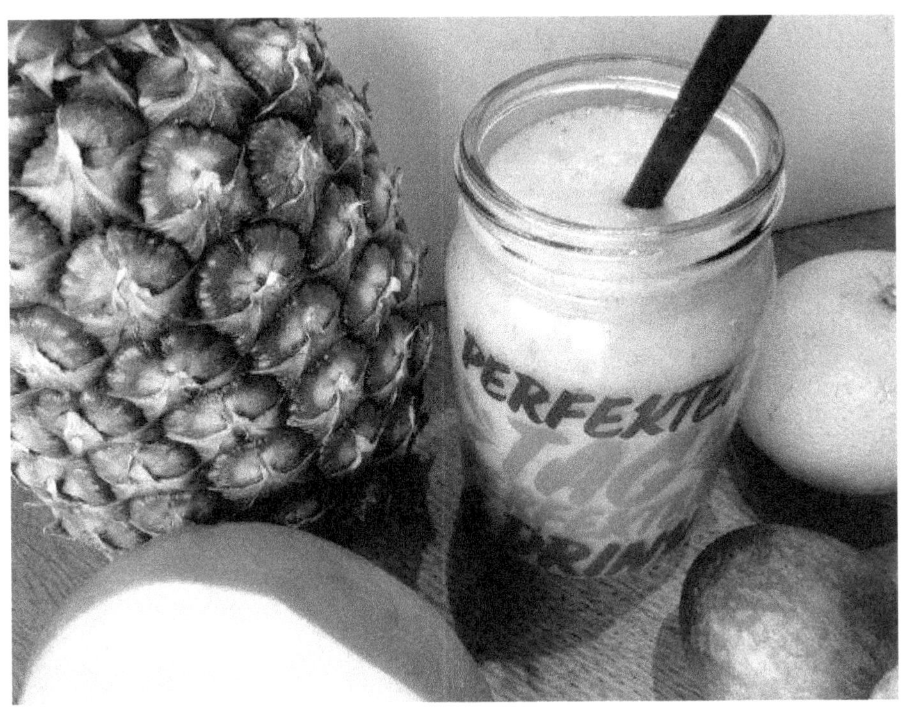

PERFEKTE
FRU...

Peanut Butter Smoothie

The ultimate protein smoothie, peanut butter is high in healthy fats and protein, and can easily be added to create a delicious smoothie. There is the option of adding cocoa powder for additional flavor, though this recipe is tasty just with the peanut butter on its own, or with a banana. Choose peanut butter with little or no salt, and without sugar, as you can add your own type of sweetener as desired. Almond or hemp milk can be added to boost the protein content, especially if you're embarking on a long jog or bicycle ride.

- 2 cups of almond or hemp milk

- 1 cup of peanut butter

- 2 tablespoons of sweetener

- 1 banana

- ¼ cups of crushed peanuts

Combine the milk, peanut butter, and sweetener into the blender and mix for 30 seconds or until smooth. Add in the banana and crushed peanuts to blend for another 20 seconds, then serve. This smoothie makes two servings and can be prepared in under six minutes.

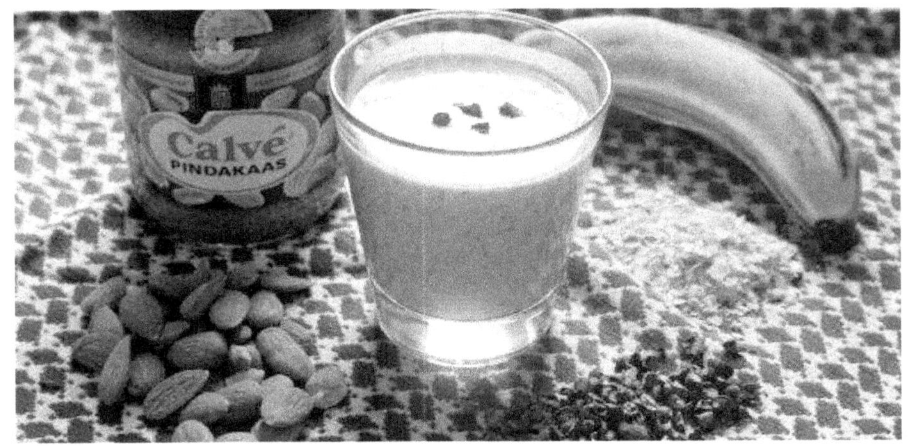
Calvé
PINDAKAAS

Tahini and Maple Syrup Smoothie

This is one of the only smoothies that does not contain fruit, though it is a decadent treat that combines the nutty flavor of tahini with the sweetness of maple syrup. A banana can be added to boost the fiber content of this recipe.

- 1 ½ cups of almond milk

- ¾ cups of tahini

- 2 tablespoons of maple syrup

- 1 banana (optional)

Combine and mix in a blender the tahini, milk, and maple syrup for a quarter of a minute. Add in the banana (if desired), extra milk as needed, and process for another 20 seconds, then serve. This recipe makes about two servings and takes about five minutes to prepare.

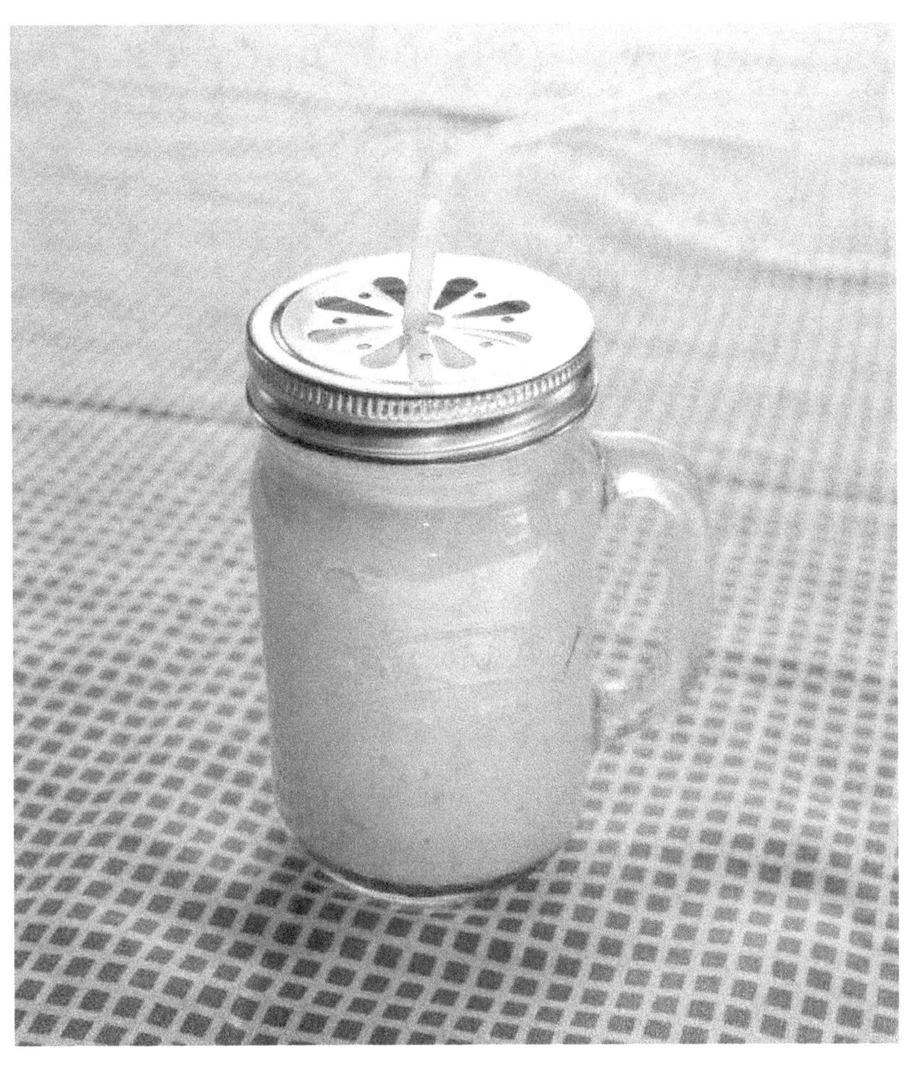

Chapter 4: 10 Soups and Salad Recipes

Five Soup Recipes

Miso Soup

A popular soup in Asian cuisine, miso soup is tasty, easy to make, and healthy. Most grocery stores and natural or specialty food stores offer dried miso in soup-making kits or as a paste that can be added to soups and sauces. Miso is available in white, yellow, and red varieties, where the white is mild in flavor (fermented over several weeks or on month), yellow is slightly stronger (several months of fermenting), and red is the strongest, most pungent flavor (several months or more – up to one year of fermentation). White and yellow are most commonly used, as their flavors are mild and easy to combine with other ingredients.

- 2-3 tablespoons miso paste

- 3-4 cups of water

- ½ cup of mushroom, sliced

- 1 cup of green onion, chopped

- 1 cup of sliced tofu (small cubes, ½-inch each)

- 1 cup of dried seaweed (nori)

In a small cooking pot, boil the water and add in the miso paste, stirring consistently for ten minutes or longer, until boiling. Add in the tofu, seaweed, and mushrooms, and continue cooking until all ingredients are tender. Serve and toss in the green onions. This soup is often served with sushi or sashimi and can also be paired with stir-fries or roasts.

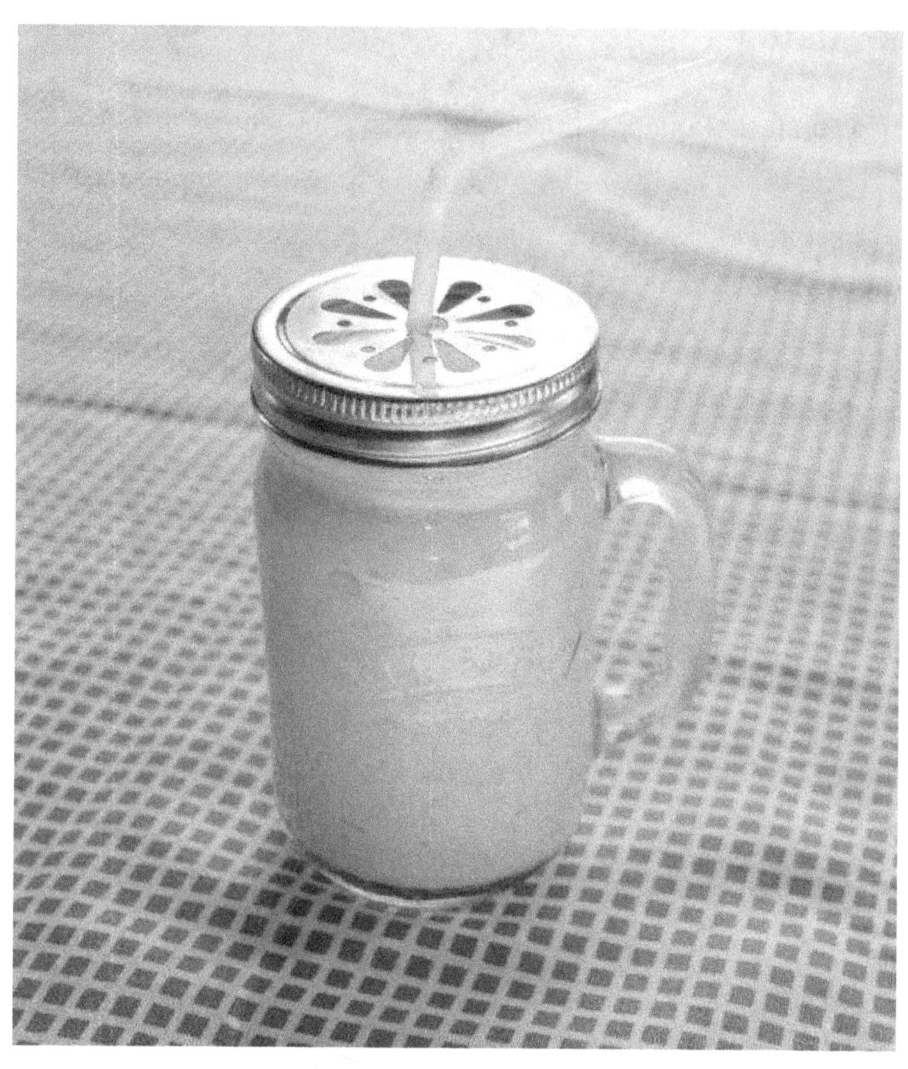

Vegetable Broth

Creating a tasty, nutritious vegetable broth is the basis for creating many delicious soups and stews. The vegan broth is readily available in most grocery stores, though it is ideal to make it from scratch, which allows you to customize the ingredients you include based on your preferences. For example, you may want to add more onion and garlic than a standard broth, as well as certain herbs and spices. Preparing a broth can take up to twenty hours to fully saturate the flavor of the vegetable into the water so that it can be strong enough to provide a base to many other soups.

To get started, choose the vegetables you want, and include peelings, peels, and leftovers from other meals to reduce the amount of waste:

- Onions, including skins

- Garlic cloves and leftover skins and feelings

- Shredded cabbage, stems, etc.

- Kale and other leafy greens (include the stems)

- Carrots

- Celery

- Bay leaves

- Dried herbs, leaves, and spices (sage, basil, etc.)

- Potato peels and skins

- Yam peels and skins

- Dried chili pepper

Pour 6-8 cups of water in a large cooking pot. The amount of water can be adjusted according to the number of vegetables and other ingredients included to ensure they are adequately covered. Add in all the ingredients (above) or a similar assortment according to preference and bring to a boil. Add sea salt and any additional spices or flavors and continue boiling for 15-20 mins. Lower the fire in the stove and gently boil for another 5-6 hours. If you need to turn off the stove, leave the pot covered and reheat later. It can take up to 20 hours to adequately transfer all the flavors to the water to make the soup base or broth. Once this is done, drain and use the broth to make other soups, or enjoy in a small bowl or cup. It will last for about a week if the broth is stored in a fridge. It will last up to 3 months if stored in the freezer.

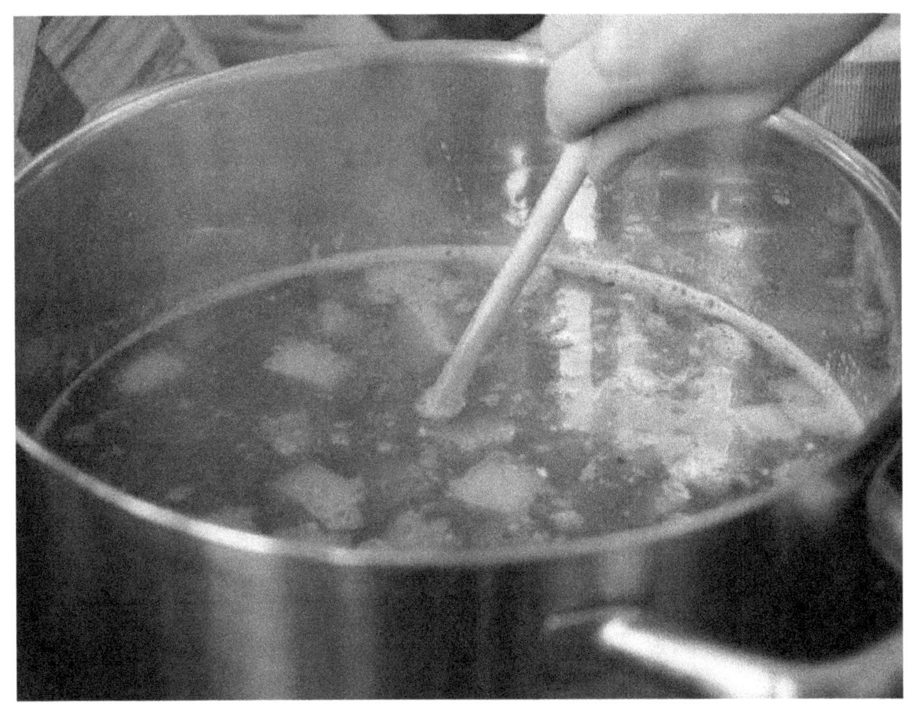

Butternut Squash Soup

This is a tasty soup that's mild and pleasant in flavor. Butternut squash is the variety used for this recipe, though any type of squash can be used if available. To prepare the squash, bake in the oven for 30 minutes whole at 375 degrees, and poke several holes with a fork to allow the inside to cook well. After 30 minutes, remove from the oven, slice in half or quarters, and bake again in almost half an hour in the same baking sheet that has been lined with parchment paper. Remove the seeds and scoop the flesh of the squash into a bowl, then set aside.

- 1 butternut squash, roasted, seeded, and flesh removed

- 4 cups of vegetable broth

- ½ cup of chopped onion

- 2 teaspoons of thyme

- 1 cup of coconut milk

- 1 teaspoon of black pepper

Bring the four cups of vegetable broth to a boil, then add in the onion, baked squash, thyme, black pepper, and coconut milk. Lower the heat and cook on medium, stirring regularly for another 15-20 minutes. Remove from the stove to cool, and process until smooth in the blender in batches. Pour the soup again in the same pot so that it can be reheated, then add more thyme, black pepper, and serve. This recipe makes approximately 4-6 servings and can take 1.5 hours to prepare (including roasting the squash).

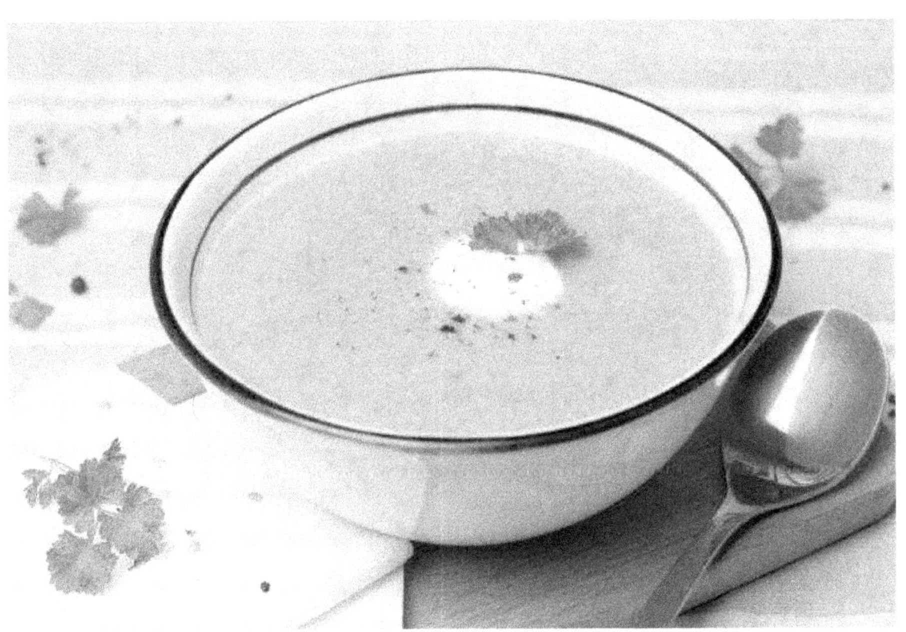

Ginger Carrot Soup

This is a tasty soup that combines the mellow, sweet taste of carrots with the strong impression of ginger for a warming soup. This recipe uses 5 cups of vegetable broth and 3 cups of sliced carrots, which may require extra preparation time to slice the carrots and make the broth unless it is store-bought.

- 2 diced onions

- 5 cups of vegetable broth

- 3-4 cups of carrots, sliced

- 2 teaspoons of ground ginger (fresh)

- 1 teaspoon of black pepper

- Dried or fresh parsley, for garnish

- 1 cup of coconut milk

- ½ cup of vegan sour cream

Cook the onions, carrots, and olive oil in a cooking pot that is large in size for about eight minutes in medium-heat setting, or until soft.

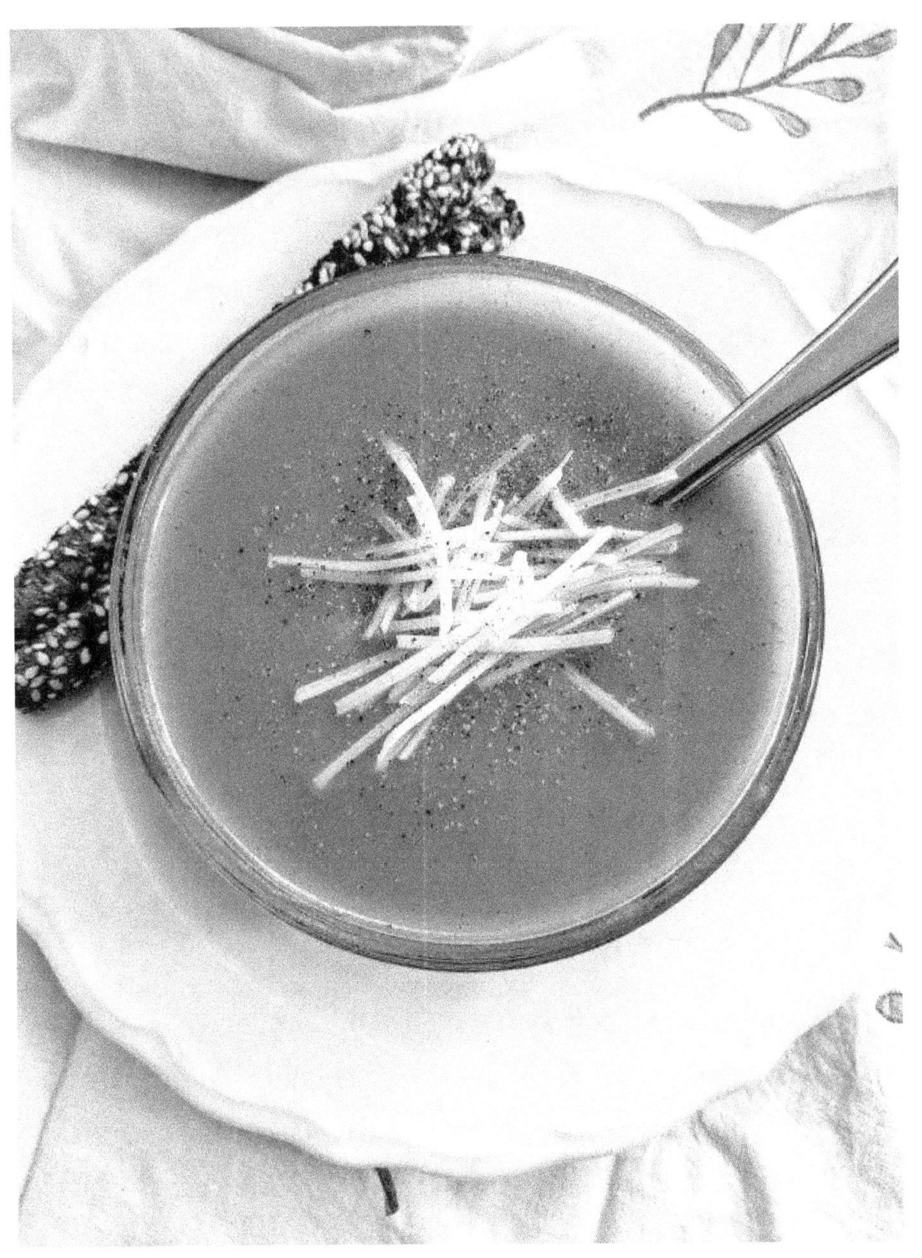

Green Pea Soup

A slightly sweet and savory dish, green pea soup is easy to prepare and makes a tasty dish in a vegan diet. Frozen or fresh peas can be used and are recommended due to their flavor (canned peas are another option, though they don't taste quite the same).

- 1 bag of frozen peas

- 2 tablespoons of olive oil

- 1 onion, chopped

- 3 cups of vegetable broth

- 1 teaspoon of dill (fresh or dried)

- 1 teaspoon of tarragon

- 1 teaspoon of black pepper

Use a large-sized pot to warm the olive oil in a stove temperature set in medium-heat. Add the onion, simmering for a couple of minutes. Pour the broth and spices (tarragon, dill, and black pepper) and continue to cook, then increase the heat so that it begins to boil. Lower the heat and add in the peas and cook on low-medium for about 10-15 minutes until peas are tender, then remove and chill. Use a food processor to pulse the soup batch by batch. Serve hot or cold. This recipe makes 4-6 servings and takes about 30 minutes.

Add a dollop of coconut yogurt or sour cream on top of the soup when serving.

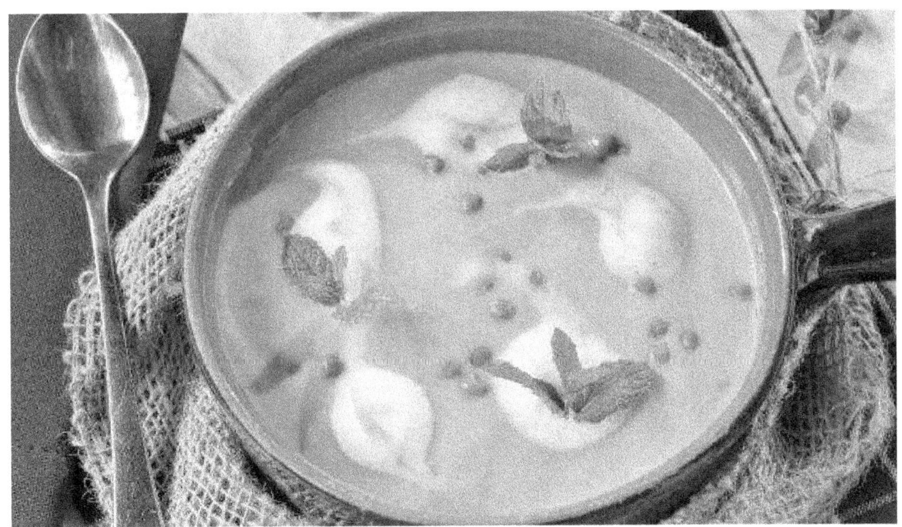

Five Salad Recipes

Salads don't have to be the boring side dishes most people consider them to be or the small handful of leaves next to the main course. Salads can be the dinner or side dish and with much more flavor and excitement than their traditional variations. Each of these recipes combines a few or more tastes that contrast and compliment at once. These are great for lunch, for a meal on-the-go, or a potluck.

Quinoa Salad

This salad is a full meal on its own, as it contains all the nutrients you need in just one serving. Quinoa makes an excellent base with a variety of fresh vegetables, herbs, nuts, and seeds.

- 1 cup of uncooked quinoa
- 1 small or medium cucumber (sliced, about one cup)
- 2 cups of water
- 2 cups of bok choy
- 1 red bell pepper, diced

- ½ cup of dried cranberries and/or blueberries

- ½ cups of mixed sunflower seeds, pumpkin seeds, crushed walnuts, pecans, and other nuts

- ½ cups of fresh parsley, dill, mint, basil, and/or cilantro

For the dressing:

- Dash of sea salt

- 1 teaspoon of maple syrup or low carb sweetener

- 2 tablespoons of apple cider vinegar

- 3 tablespoons of olive oil

- Dash of black pepper

- 2 tablespoons of lemon juice (freshly squeezed)

In preparing the dressing, you need to put together first and mix all the ingredients for the dressing in a small mixing container before setting it aside. Combine the salad ingredients and toss evenly, then serve with the vinaigrette. This dish makes about 4-6 servings and takes about 15-20 minutes to prepare.

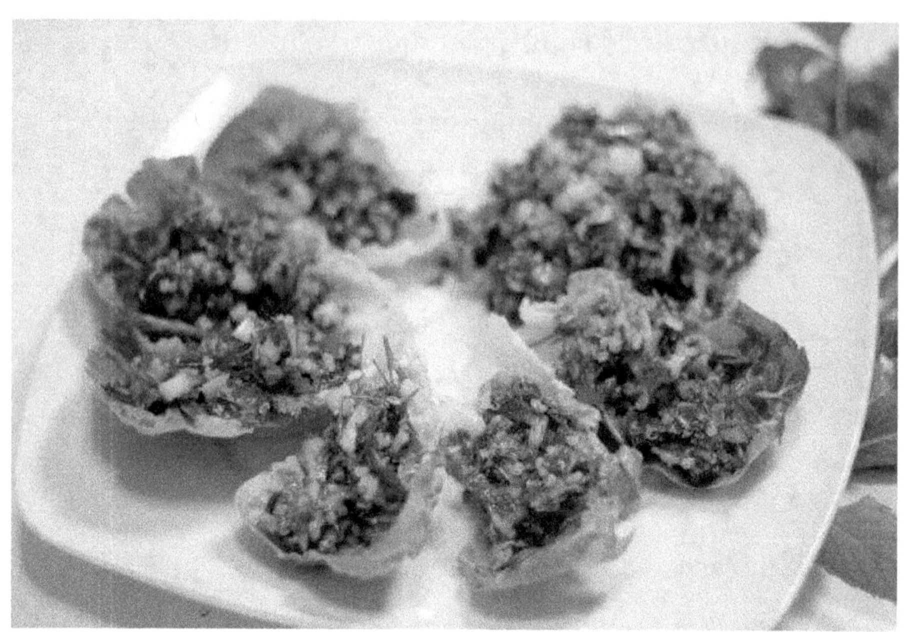

Kale Blueberry Salad

Kale is a superfood that contains a healthy dose of calcium, protein, fiber, and antioxidants. It's a bitter-tasting vegetable that compliments a wide range of flavors, sweet, spicy, and savory. This salad gives kale a lift with a sweet infusion of blueberries and a three-ingredient vinaigrette.

- 1 cup of fresh blueberries

- ½ cups of sliced almonds

- 1 bunch of kale (stems removed, sliced or shredded)

For the dressing:

- 1 teaspoon of maple syrup

- 2 tablespoons of lime or lemon juice

- 2 teaspoons of olive oil

Mix the three ingredients for the vinaigrette in a mixing dish that is small in size before setting it aside. In a larger bowl, combine the sliced kale, and toss in the fresh blueberries. Serve sprinkled with the vinaigrette and topped with sliced almonds.

There are a few variations to consider for this salad:

- Lightly toast the almond slices in a skillet for one minute before topping

- Use 1 teaspoon of blueberry marmalade instead of maple syrup for the dressing

Note: There are many types of kale to choose from (red, curly, black kale) and all or any if they are suitable for this salad.

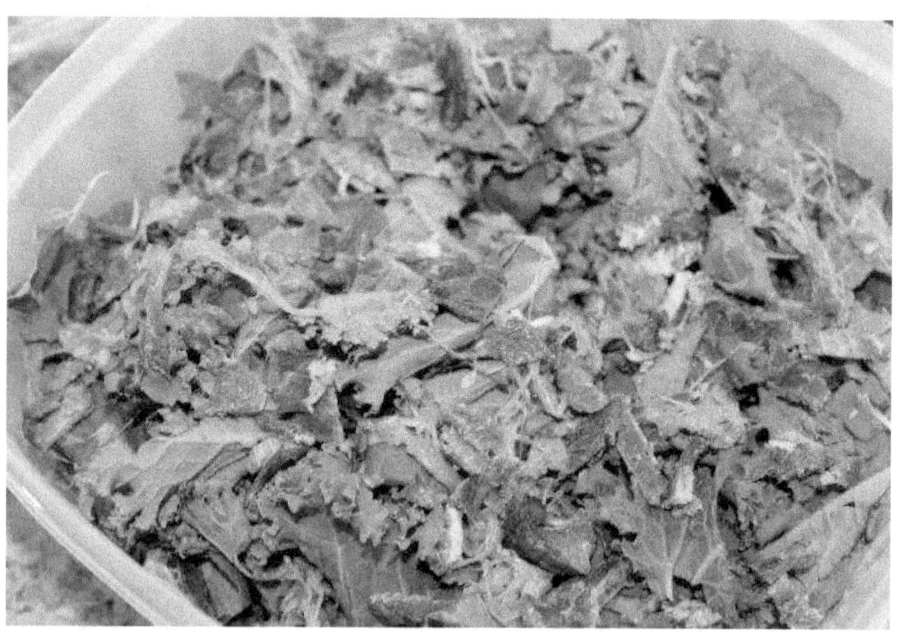

Spinach, Mandarin, and Walnut Salad

Spinach is an excellent source of iron and calcium. Combined with mandarin and walnuts, there's a good source of vitamins and fiber as well. The dressing used for this salad adds a citrus flavor and maple syrup.

- 1 bunch of spinach, washed and drained

- 3-4 mandarins, peeled and pieces (slices) removed

- 1 cup of coarsely chopped walnuts

- ½ cup of shredded carrots

For the dressing:

- 2 teaspoons of olive oil

- 3 teaspoons of orange juice (freshly squeezed)

- 1 teaspoon of maple syrup

Mix the ingredients for the salad dressing in a small bowl and set aside. In a larger bowl, add the fresh spinach (washed and drained in a colander), and toss in the shredded carrots, walnuts, and mandarin slices. Serve with dressing. This recipe makes approximately 4-5 servings and can be prepared within 15 minutes.

Arugula and Roasted Pear Salad

This recipe features a roasted pear, which adds a naturally mellow and sweet flavor to the arugula and other ingredients. Pecans and walnuts are added to balance the texture and flavors. Crumbled vegan cheese can also be added as a topping, if available.

- ½ cups chopped walnuts

- 1 cup of coarsely chopped pecans

- 2 cups of chopped arugula

- 1 roasted pear, sliced in half

For the dressing:

- 1 teaspoon of maple syrup

- 2 teaspoons of lime juice

- 2 teaspoons of olive oil

To roast the pear, set the oven to 350, slice the pear in half, and place face down on a baking sheet prepared with a parchment paper. Bake for half an hour, then remove and cool for 10-15 minutes. Mix the dressing ingredients together well, then set aside. Combine all the salad items and blend evenly. Lightly coat with dressing and serve.

Options for this salad include the following:

- Add ½ cup of dried cranberries

- Sliced coconut chips (approx. ¼ cup)

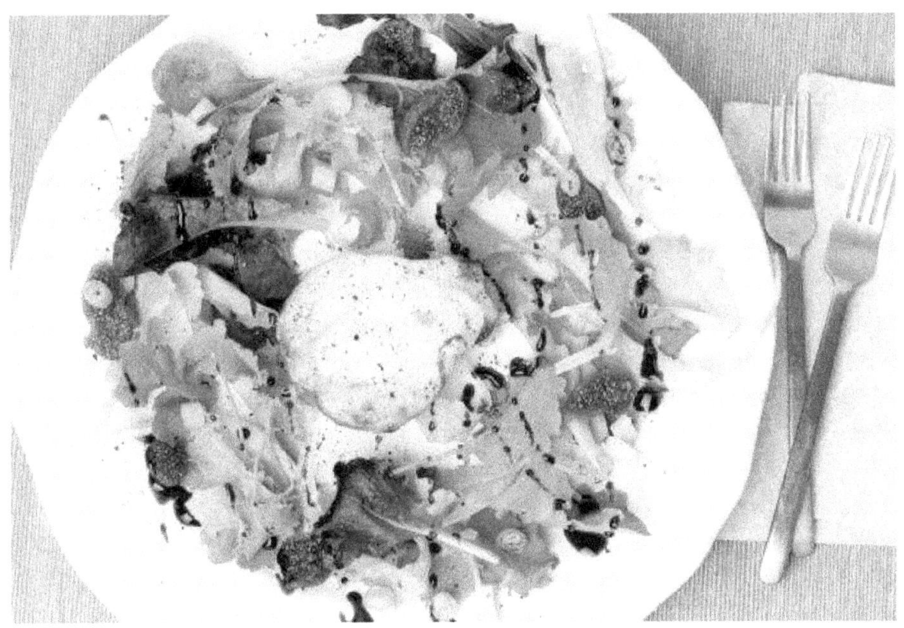

<u>***Fruit Salad***</u>

This is a fun and effortless salad to prepare, which includes adding and combining the fruit options of your choice. When selecting fruits, make sure they are fresh and in season. Frozen fruit can be used, though it would need to thaw first, and may not have the same texture (berries are the best option if frozen fruit is used). The list below is a suggested combination of fruits to include in this recipe:

- 1 large apple, sliced (skin can be removed or left on)

- 1-2 mandarins, peeled and broken apart into slices/pieces or one large orange, sliced and skin removed

- 1 cup of grapes (seedless)

- 1 cup of sliced cantaloupe or honeydew into cubes

- 1 cup of sliced watermelon

- ½ cup of sliced strawberries stems removed

- ½ cup of blueberries

- ½ cup of raspberries

- 1 cup of sliced pineapples

This salad is easy to prepare and may include as little or as many of the fruits above (and more). Wash, chop, and assemble all fruits and drain in a colander. Serve with freshly squeezed lemon and garnish with fresh mint leaves. The salad serves 4-6 and takes approximately 15-20 minutes to prepare.

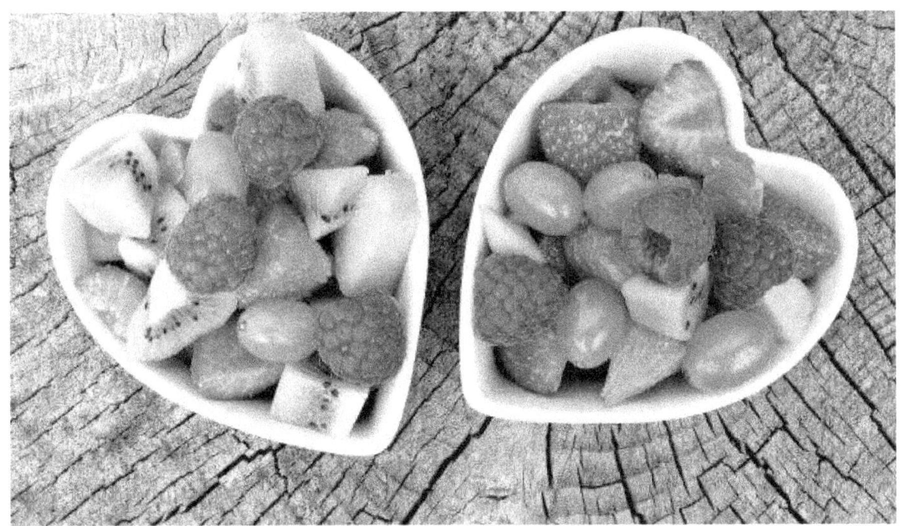

Chapter 5: 10 Main Dish Recipes

Main Meal Recipes and Sides

There are many options for vegan dinners, both the main feature and the side dishes. Tofu and tempeh often play a central role in main dishes, though many pulses and vegetables, including grains, can take center stage as well. The following recipes focus on several options that can be varied, whether your focus is tofu or tempeh, beans, or a wide range of vegetables in one dish.

Lentil Dal

One of the most popular Indian dishes, lentil dal is an excellent choice for many reasons: it's high in fiber, protein, and calcium. Turmeric, a spice used in this recipe, contains high amounts of antioxidants and fights inflammation in the body. This dish can be prepared mild, or with some added spice. Any lentils can be used, though red lentils are best, as they cook easily and mix well with the other ingredients.

- 1 green chili pepper, diced (with stem removed)

- 1 cup of diced onion (white or yellow)

- 1 tablespoon of olive oil

- 2 teaspoons of cumin seeds

- 1 cup of red lentils

- 1 teaspoon of cinnamon

- 4 crushed garlic cloves

- 2 teaspoons of grated ginger (fresh is recommended)

- 1 small or medium tomato, diced

- 1 teaspoon of paprika

- ½ teaspoon of cardamom

- 1 teaspoon of turmeric

- 1 teaspoon of sea salt

- 1 teaspoon of lemon juice

- 1 teaspoon of chili powder (optional)

- 1 cup of chopped parsley or cilantro leaves

If using dried lentils, rinse and bring to a boil in a saucepan covered in water, reduce, and cook on medium for 15-20 minutes. While the lentils are cooking, let a skillet heat up before adding the olive oil, cumin, and cinnamon on medium for five minutes, then add in the garlic, onion, green chili, chili powder (optional ingredient), and ginger. Simmer for another five or six minutes, then add the following items: salt, tomatoes, paprika, cardamom, and turmeric. Continue to cook for another five minutes. When the lentils are cooked, drain and stir in the skillet mixed with the lentils, combining evenly. Add fresh lemon juice. Serve with cilantro or parsley leaves.

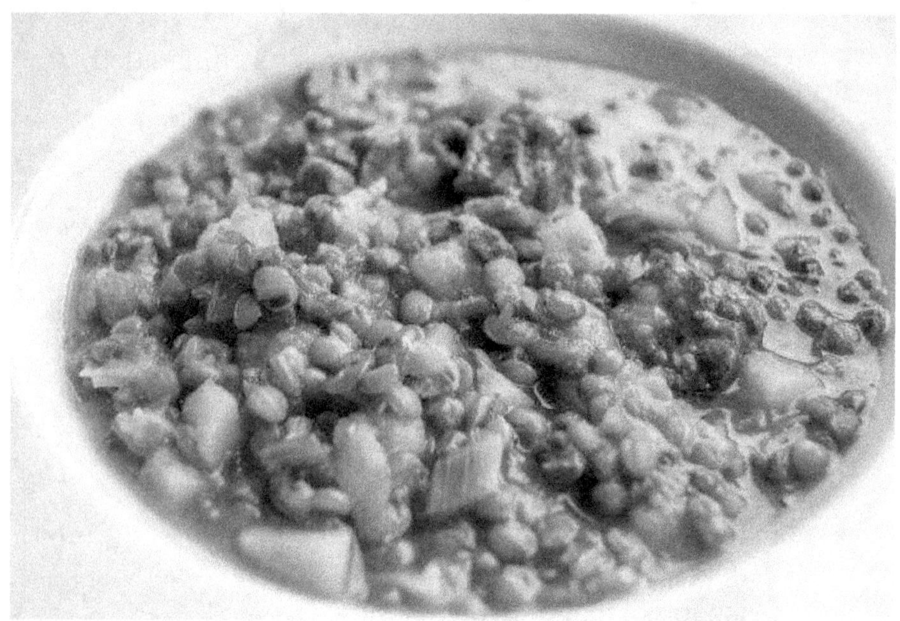

Tofu Bake with Squash

This recipe is basically two sides in one to create a nourishing meal. Squash bakes well alongside tofu, and both are done within the same time frame, which makes this an easy meal to prepare. The only additional preparation for the tofu involves marinating in the following three ingredients:

- ½ cup of olive oil

- 1 cup of soy sauce (use low sodium, if you require less salt in your diet)

- 2 teaspoons of sesame oil (optional)

- 2 tablespoons of lemon juice

Combine all the above ingredients in a bowl and set aside. Rinse and drain one package (or block) of firm tofu and set aside in a small or medium food keeper. The tofu should be covered with the marinade. Place in the refrigerate for two hours at a minimum. When the tofu is ready, drain and retain ½ cups of the liquid and set aside. Heat in an oven to 350. In a baking dish of medium size, lay the marinated tofu and place two halves of a squash beside the tofu (if there isn't enough room, use two baking dishes; one for the tofu and one for the squash.) Pour the ½ cup of retained liquid from the marinade over the tofu, and if desired, coat in sesame seeds. Bake with the squash for 35-45 minutes, until the tofu is slightly crispy, and the squash is tender inside.

This dish makes about 4-6 servings and works well with a dark leafy green salad or cooked spinach. A small bowl of miso soup makes an excellent side, or a slightly thicker version of a miso-based soup can be poured over the squash before serving.

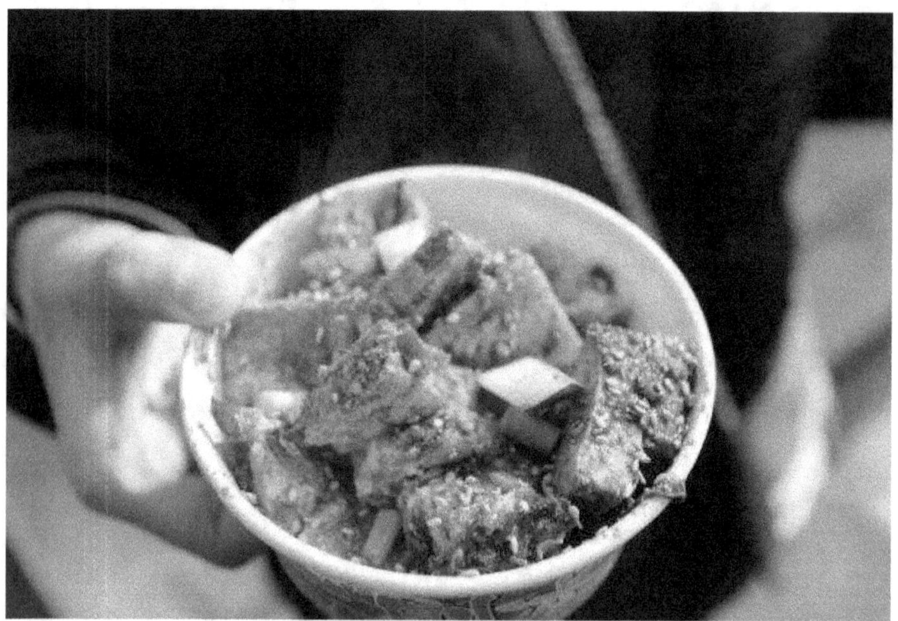

Sweet and Sour Tempeh Skillet

Tempeh is fermented soy food which a strong, textured taste similar to meat. Like tofu, tempeh takes on the flavors of other foods it is cooked with, and marinating is one of the best methods of getting the most out of tempeh. In this recipe, a sweet and sour marinade is prepared by combining the following ingredients and covering one block of tempeh (sliced into cubes) and refrigerated for two hours:

- 3 tablespoons of olive oil

- ½ cup of orange or pineapple juice

- 1 teaspoon of maple syrup

- 3 teaspoons of vinegar (white wine vinegar)

- 2 teaspoons soy sauce

Mix these ingredients thoroughly in a small bowl, then cover the tempeh in a sealed container and chill for a minimum of two hours.

The skillet meal consists of the following ingredients:

- ½ cup of pineapple, cut into small cubes

- 1 clove of garlic, diced

- 1 red onion, diced

- 1 block of marinated tempeh (as shown above)

- ½ cup of snow peas

- ½ cup of chopped celery

- ½ cup of sliced carrots

- 1 or 2 bell peppers, sliced

- 2 teaspoons ground ginger

- 2 teaspoons of soy sauce

- 2 tablespoons of olive oil

Heat the skillet on medium heat with olive oil. Add and sauté the onion and garlic. Continue cooking it for a couple of minutes. In the meantime, remove the tempeh and drain, retaining ½ cup of the liquid. Add the tempeh and liquid to the skillet and cook for ten mins, then add in the rest of the ingredients before continuing to gently boil on low or medium for another 10-15 minutes, until the vegetables are cooked but still crispy. Remove from heat and serve with rice or noodles.

Some variations to consider for this recipe include the following:

- Sprinkle with raw or lightly toasted sesame seeds

- Add a couple of teaspoons of crushed peanuts as a topping

- Serve with fresh sliced pineapple instead of or in addition to the cooked version included in this recipe.

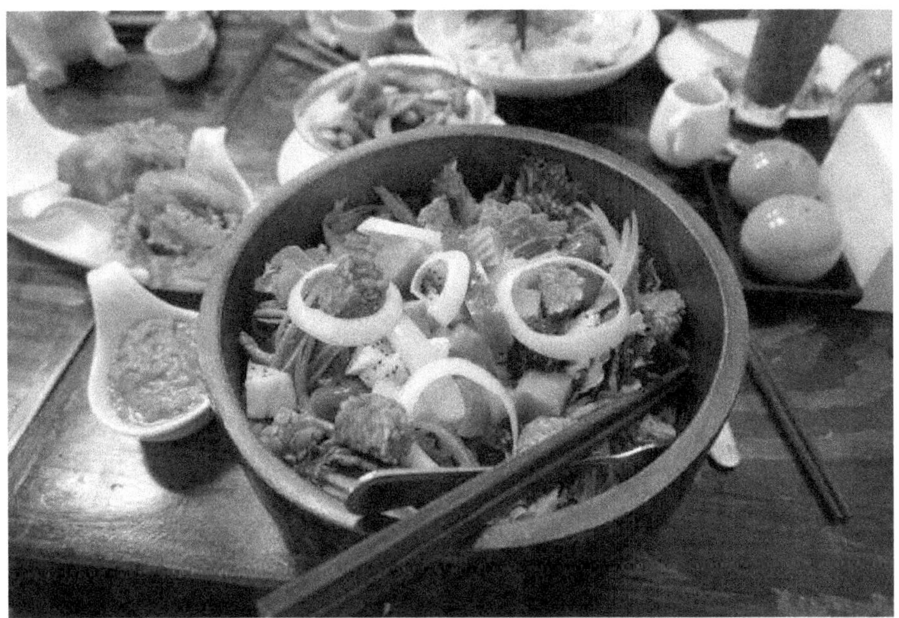

Veggie Skillet Dinner

This dish is full of nutrients, including dome leafy greens to increase your intake of iron and calcium. If you want to explore a wide variety of textures, flavors, and combinations, this is an opportunity to mix a lot of options together. For this dish, it's advantageous to use a large wok or similarly sized skillet to contain a large volume of vegetables. Consider adding all or some of the following:

Vegetables:

- Snow peas
- Carrots
- Celery
- Bok choy
- Broccoli
- Cauliflower
- Bell peppers
- Green chilies
- Bean sprouts

- Mushrooms (any variety – shitake, Portobello, or button mushrooms)

- Baby corn

- Onions (white, red, or yellow)

- Garlic

- Chopped raw spinach

- Kale leaves, chopped

Herbs and leaves:

- Basil leaves

- Parsley

- Tarragon

- Bay leaves

- Curry spice or leaves

Other ingredients:

- Soy sauce

- Teriyaki sauce

- Sesame seeds

- Sliced almonds

- Mandarin slices or pineapple chunks

Heat the wok or large skillet on medium and add olive oil, followed by teriyaki or soy sauce (chili or curry paste are also options), then add the desired herbs and spices and continue to simmer. Add in the vegetables that take the longest to cook first: celery, carrots, broccoli, cauliflower, etc. and cook for 10-15 minutes before adding the remaining ingredients, leaving the mushrooms and bean sprouts last, as they fry quickly. Sprinkle with nuts and/or leaves. Serve with mandarin or pineapple chunks, if preferred, or add them in while cooking (or omit completely).

There are some interesting variations: add tamarind for a Phad Thai-style flavor and serve with noodles or mix the soy sauce and olive oil with 1-2 tablespoons of peanut butter for a thicker sauce for the stir fry.

Chickpea Curry

A warm, aromatic dish, chickpea curry is an excellent meal that can be enjoyed alone, or with a small, simple side such as a salad or soup. This dish is prepared with coconut milk, which is often used as a base for curries, as it enhances the flavor and works well with garlic, onions, chili as well as a variety of species and ingredients.

- 1 large can or 1 ½ small cans of chickpeas, drained and rinsed

- 1 medium or large red onion, sliced

- 4 crushed cloves of garlic

- 2 tablespoons of grated ginger (fresh)

- 1 tablespoon of garam masala

- 1 teaspoon of black pepper

- 1 teaspoon of turmeric

- 1 large can of coconut milk, or 2 cups

- 2 cups of diced tomatoes

- 1 teaspoon of sea salt

- ½ teaspoon of cayenne pepper or chili powder

- 1 tablespoon of lemon or lime juice

- 1 cup of sliced cilantro leaves

- 2 tablespoons of olive oil

In a medium-sized skillet, let the olive oil heated before adding the garlic, salt, and red onion. Cook for a few minutes, then add in the ginger and cook another two minutes. Mix in the turmeric, black pepper, garam masala, cayenne pepper or chili powder, and tomatoes. Simmer for another 5-10 minutes, then gently pour in the coconut milk before lowering the heat. Cook on medium-low and stir continuously until coconut milk and all ingredients are done. Test taste and season with additional flavors if needed, before serving. This dish serves up to 6 people and can be served with basmati rice or rice noodles.

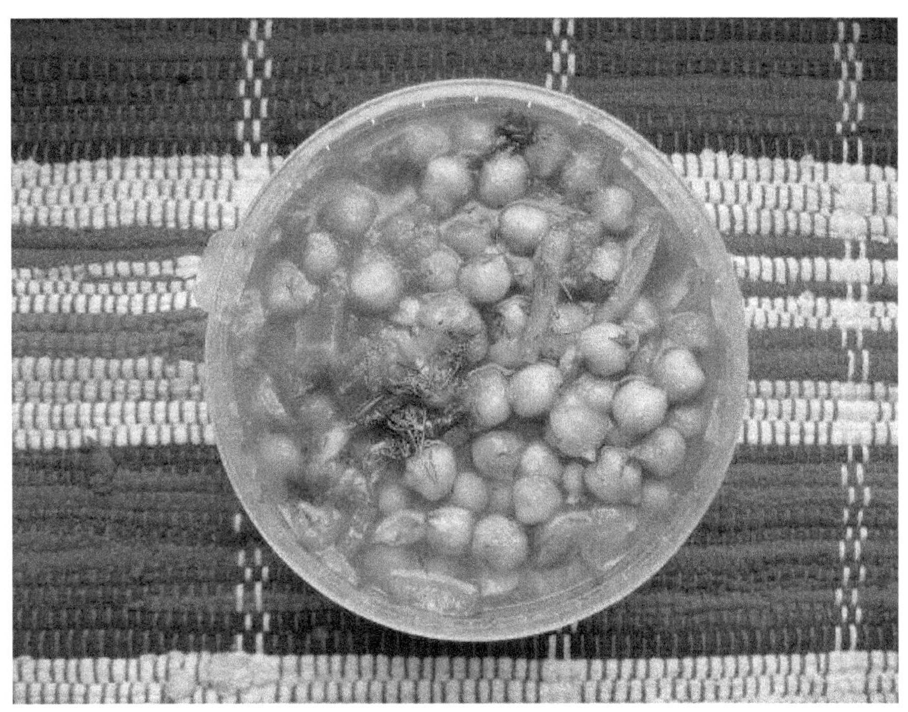

Vegan Chili

During the colder months, chili is a hearty and filling meal that is inexpensive to prepare and easy to make. There are some options to explore with this meal, including the types of beans, spices, and vegetables to include. For added protein, TVP (textured vegetable protein) can be added. This is a supplement available in dried form, found in natural food or bulk stores. It is used as a quick and effortless way to add a quick dose of protein to soups, stews, and other recipes for vegan meals.

- 2 large cans or 4-5 cups of diced tomatoes (or the same portion of fresh, sliced tomatoes)
- 1 ½ cups of tomato paste
- 4 crushed cloves of garlic
- 1 sliced onion (medium)
- 1 can of kidney beans (white or red)
- 1 can of chickpeas
- 1 can of black beans
- 1 can of pinto beans
- 1 cup of sliced carrots
- 1 cup of diced celery

- ½ cup of sliced mushrooms

- 3-4 tablespoons of chili powder

- 2 teaspoons of black pepper

- 2 jalapeno peppers, sliced

- 1 teaspoon of sea salt

- 1 tablespoon ground cumin

- 1 cup of fresh cilantro or parsley, chopped

- 2 tablespoons of textured vegetable protein (optional, only use for extra protein)

- 2 tablespoons of olive oil

- 1 cup shredded vegan cheese (optional)

Use a cooking pot of large size in heating up the olive oil before adding the chili pepper, garlic, black pepper, cumin, sea salt, and other spices. Cook on medium for 5 minutes, before adding the vegetables and sautéing for another six mins. Add in the tomatoes and paste, stirring and mixing the spices into the sauce. Drain and rinse all the beans and return it back inside the pot. Cook, stirring, for about fifteen mins in medium-heat setting, then reduce and cook for another hour, adding more spices as desired. Serve topped with cilantro or parsley, and/or vegan cheese (shredded).

Soy ground round or other vegan versions of ground "beef" can be added to thicken the chili, or in place of the textured vegetable protein, if used at all.

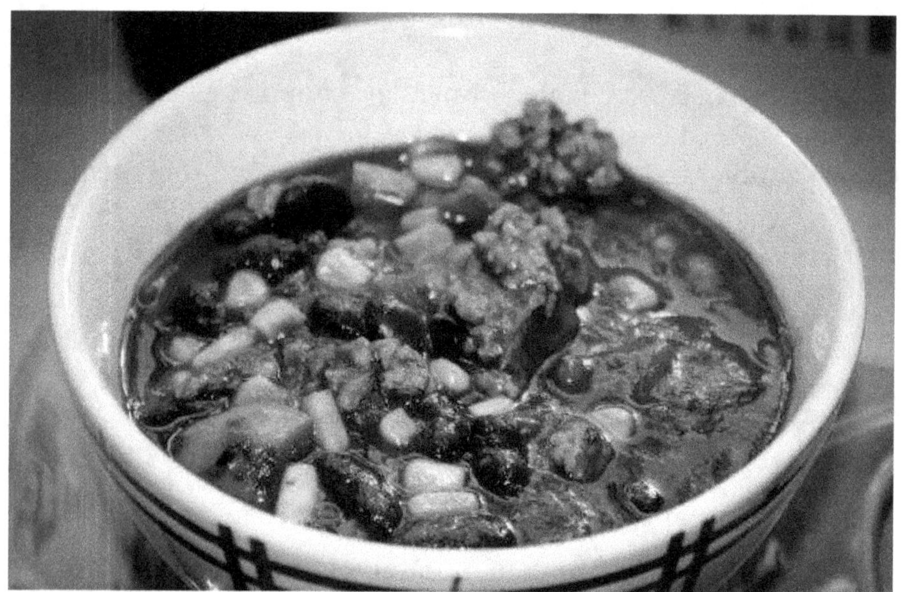

Spaghetti with Sauce and Baked Zucchini

A twist on a regular spaghetti and meat sauce dish, this meal uses baked zucchini as the central feature, served with the pasta sauce and noodles.

- 2 large zucchinis, sliced in half lengthwise

- 2 cans of crushed tomatoes

- ¼ cup of tomato paste

- 3 cloves of garlic, grated or crushed

- 1 teaspoon of black pepper

- 1 teaspoon of thyme

- 1 teaspoon of chili pepper

- 1 tablespoon of oregano

- Dash of sea salt

- ½ package of uncooked pasta noodles (spaghetti is recommended)

- ½ cup of vegan parmesan

Slice and rinse the zucchini, coat lightly in sea salt, and place on a baking dish lined with paper and in an oven that is already preheated to 350 degrees. Bake for 25-30 minutes. While the zucchini is in the oven, heat a medium or small skillet with olive oil and add in the oregano, chili pepper, black pepper, thyme, and sea salt. Cook for another 5-6 minutes, then add in the crushed garlic for a few more minutes until softened. Pour in the tomato paste and crushed tomatoes and reduce heat. Transfer to a large or medium cooking pot to continue stewing, if needed. In a separate cooking pot, boil up to four cups of water before adding in the pasta. Add 1 teaspoon of salt, reduce to medium, and cook until tender. Drain the spaghetti and set aside.

When the zucchini is baked, removed from the oven and place on a large oval serving dish. Scoop the spaghetti or pasta and add around the zucchini, then pour the pasta sauce over everything. Coat the top in vegan parmesan and serve. This dish serves 4-6 people and takes approximately one hour to prepare.

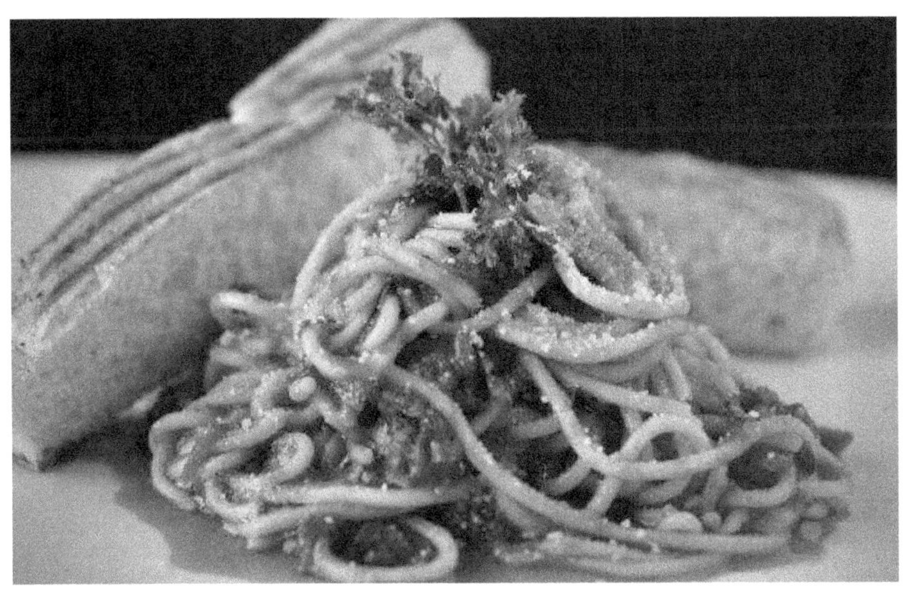

Veggie Burger Patties

If you crave burgers, these patties will provide the right fix. Served with or without a bun, these veggie burger patties can be a tasty meal on their own or as a traditional hamburger. The making of this recipe combines beans and mushrooms for a delicious mix.

- 1 small white or yellow onion, diced

- 3 green onions, sliced

- 1 teaspoon of cumin

- 1 cup of sliced mushrooms

- 1 tablespoon of olive oil

- 2 crushed cloves of garlic

- 1 cup of pinto beans

- 1 teaspoon of black pepper

- 1 teaspoon of dill or parsley

The olive oil should be heated first in a cooking pan before adding the garlic and the onions. Simmer on medium for 3-4 minutes. Add in the cumin, green onions, and mushrooms and continue to cook for another 5-6 minutes, or until the vegetables are tender. Reduce the heat to low to simmer, then remove from heat and set aside. Drain and rinse a can of pinto beans. Pour into a medium bowl and mash until they resemble refried beans. Beans can also be processed in a blender until smooth. Return the beans to the bowl and mix in the mushroom and onion mix from the skillet. Blend until smooth, then form into burger-sized patties and set aside. Heat a skillet on medium with olive oil. Lightly fry each side of each burger for about 3-4 minutes, or until browned, then serve.

Variations to this recipe include the following:

- Add one or two tablespoons of chili powder to make it spicy or one diced jalapeno pepper

- Replace pinto beans with black beans for a different taste, or combine both into the same portion

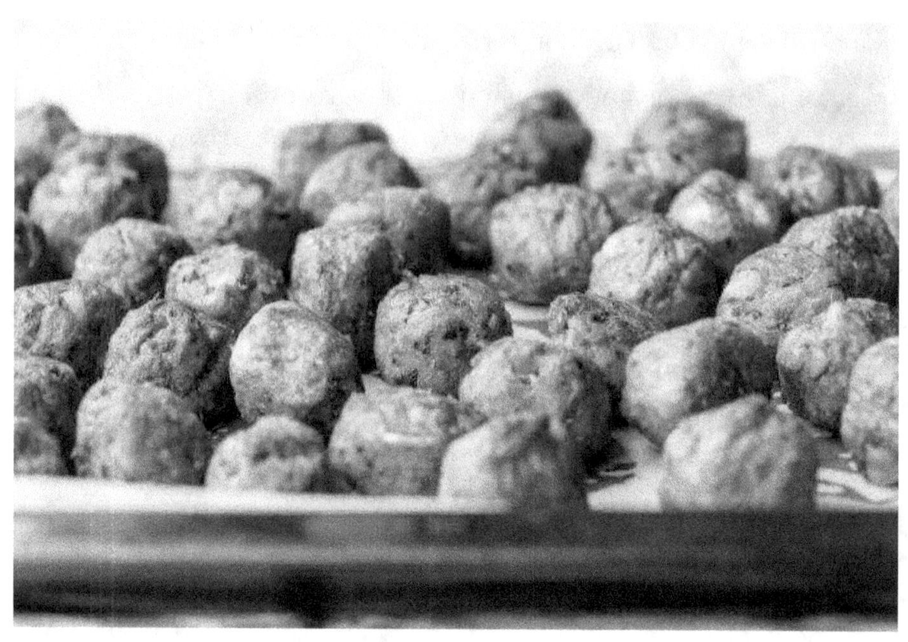

Tofu Scramble with Greens

This dish is often prepared for breakfast, though it can be prepared for any meal of the day. Firm tofu is marinated in a light broth and prepared the next morning. As with most marinades, the minimum recommended time to soak the tofu is two hours. The tofu can be prepared the night before and marinated overnight or two hours before your next meal. The ingredients are simple and easy to use:

- 1 teaspoon of black pepper

- 1 tablespoon of turmeric

- 1 teaspoon of sea salt

- 2 cups of vegetable broth

- ½ teaspoon of oregano

- ½ teaspoon of thyme

- ¼ teaspoon of tarragon

Combine the above ingredients in a small bowl to create the marinade. Drain and rinse one block of tofu and slice into cubes. Add to a small or medium container and pour the broth marinade to coat the tofu completely. If tofu is not completely covered, add more vegetable broth until it's submerged. Place in

the refrigerator for two hours or longer, then rinse and retain ½
cup of the liquid in a small bowl.

To prepare the tofu, heat a skillet on medium with olive oil.
Mash the tofu in a bowl until it is crumbly, then pour the ½ cup
of leftover liquid and mix. Add to the skillet and fry. Sprinkle
any spices you prefer, such as chili pepper, curry, and/or thyme.
To add in the greens, choose spinach or arugula (one cup), then
drain and rinse. Chop and add to the skillet. Continue to cook
until tofu is gold or browned and greens are soft, then serve.

This is an excellent dish to get as many nutrients as possible
with just a few ingredients. For a different twist on this dish,
consider the following:

- Mix two tablespoons of coconut milk with one tablespoon
  of curry powder and mix it into the tofu scramble.

- Add two tablespoons of tomato paste and a few black
  beans. Serve with salsa and sliced avocado.

- Add a sliced jalapeno or green chili for a very spicy dish,
  then serve with vegan sour cream.

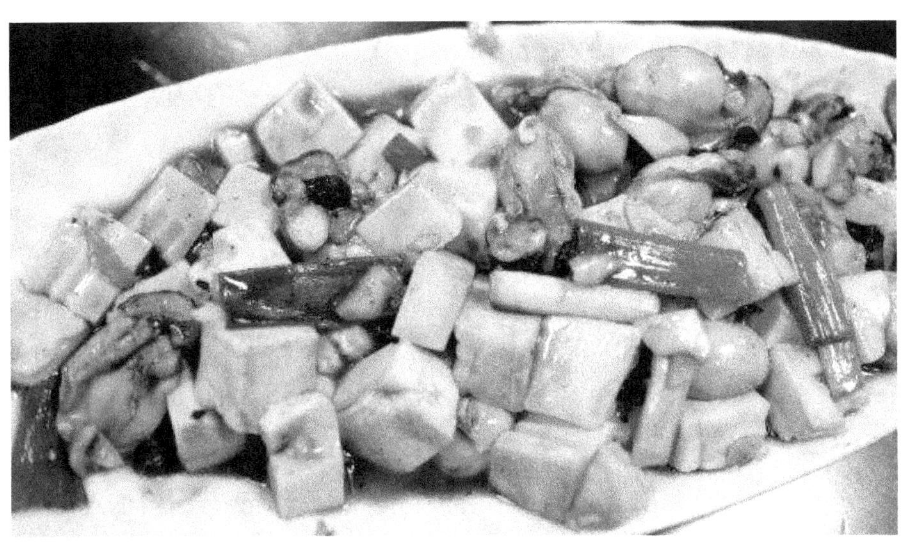

Chapter 6: 10 Snack Recipes

A vegan diet doesn't have to skip on snacks and tasty treats. There are plenty of plant-based ingredients that combine to make a wonderful assortment of bars, bite-sized treats. Consider some of the following recipes for planning your day. Packing one or two options will curb your temptation to choose sugary, high-fat snacks often offered in coffee shops and grocery stores.

Energy Bars

High protein and energy with low sugar and healthy fats, these bars are ideal to prepare for a workout or a busy day at the office. To make these bars, no baking or cooking is required. Chia seeds are an important ingredient, as they contain a wealth of nutrients, including fiber, protein, and antioxidants.

- 1 cup of pitted and sliced dates

- ½ cup of cocoa powder

- ½ cup of chia seeds

- 1 cup of crushed pistachios

- ½ cup of shredded coconut

- 1 teaspoon vanilla extract

- ½ cup of raw dark chocolate chips

- ¾ cups of raw oats

Use a food processor to smoothly blend the dates before adding the walnuts and continuing to blend. Pour the remaining items to pulse together until they are all evenly mixed. Remove and transfer the dough mixture to a small bowl and knead together, forming small, bar-shaped portions, and place on a lined baking tray. Place in the freezer for a minimum of two hours or overnight, then remove, slice, and serve.

These are delicious snacks and pack a lot of nutrients into each bite. To vary the recipe for a slightly different taste, consider the following options:

- Add 1 teaspoon of cinnamon or nutmeg

- Mix in 1 teaspoon of coconut oil

- Replace the pistachios with crushed walnuts, pecans, or slivered almonds

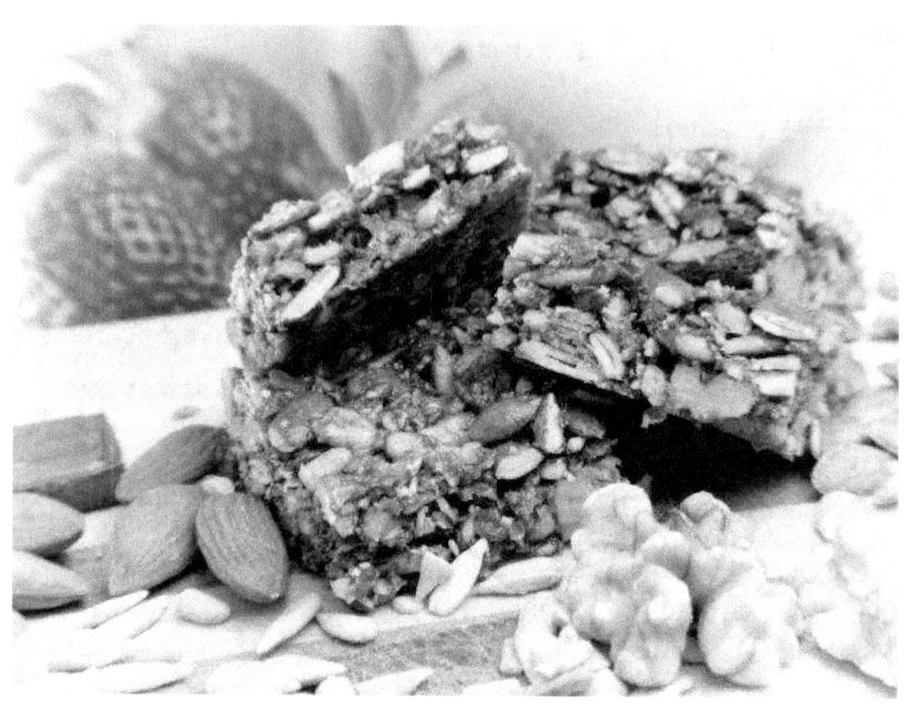

Peanut Butter and Chocolate Energy Bites

These are easy to make and minimal ingredient treats that are rolled into small, ball-sized servings. Usually, two or three can satisfy as a tasty snack in between meals. These are prepared using a small ice cube tray or silicone molds to form and freeze. No baking or cooking is required.

- 1 cup of peanut butter (sugar-free and unsalted)

- 2 tablespoons of raw oats

- 2 teaspoons of chia seeds

- 1 teaspoon of vanilla extract

- 2 tablespoons of cocoa powder

- 1 teaspoon of maple syrup

In a mixing dish of medium size, mix the peanut butter with the maple syrup until evenly mixed. Add in the cocoa powder and vanilla extra, mashing until the cocoa is completely coating the peanut butter mix, then add in the raw oats and chia seeds, using your hands to completely combine the ingredients. Form the dough into balls and add to silicone molds or an ice cube tray and freeze for one hour, then move the refrigerator. These treats can be kept up to one week in the refrigerator or a month in the freezer. This recipe makes about 4-5 servings and takes only 5-6 minutes to prepare.

For a slight variation, replace the peanut butter with tahini or almond butter. If replacing with tahini, adding a teaspoon of raw or toasted sesame seeds is another option.

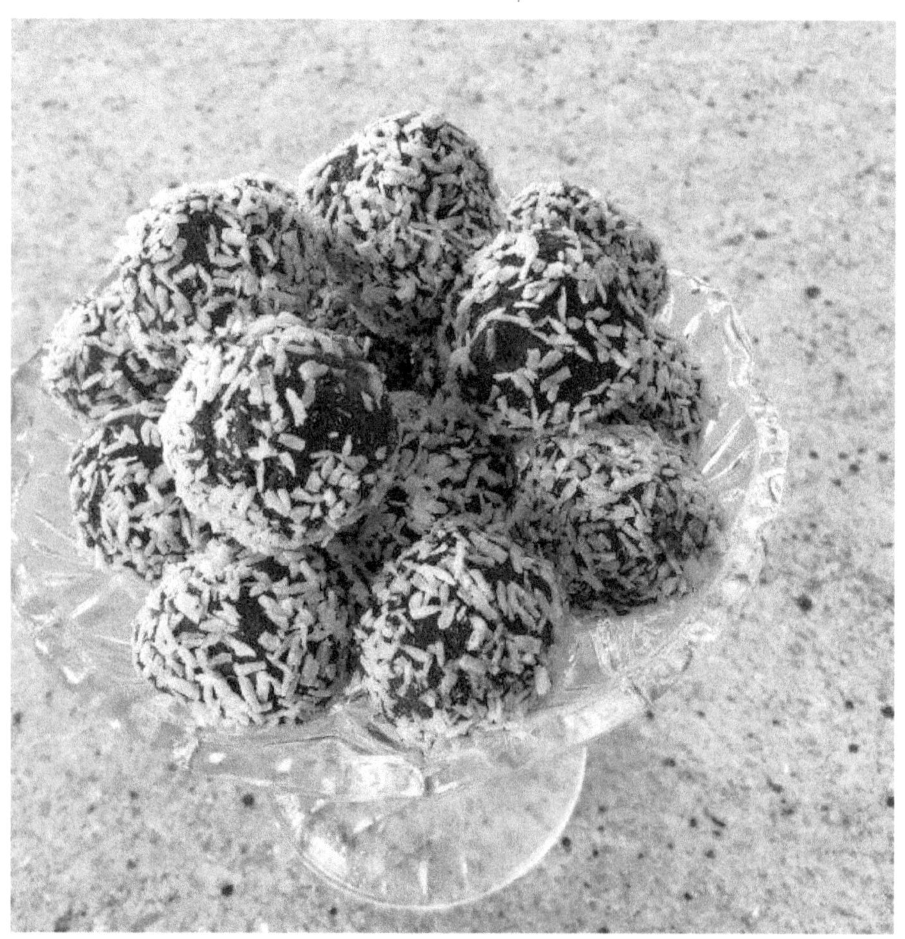

Pistachio and Cardamom Treats

This treat is created like fat bombs, which are healthy fat treats infused with a large selection or combination of flavors. In this recipe, cardamom and pistachios are combined with coconut oil to create small, bite-sized fat bombs, which are stored in the freezer for two hours before serving.

- 3 tablespoons of coconut oil, melted at room temperature

- ½ teaspoons crushed cardamom pods or powder

- 1 teaspoon of maple syrup

- 2-3 tablespoons of crushed pistachios

Blend the entire ingredients together into a small bowl and pour into silicone molds or an ice cube tray. Freeze for at least two hours before servings. Keep frozen until ready to serve. This recipe makes enough for 4-5.

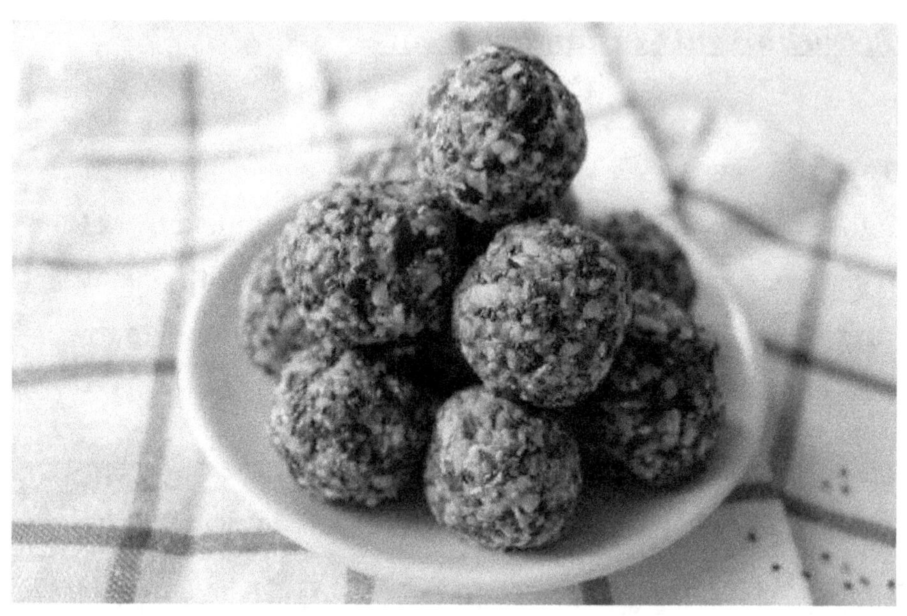

Lemon-Lime Cheesecake Cupcake Fat Bombs

Inspired by key lime pie and cheesecake, this vegan version and fat bomb version is tasty and much easier to make.

- 1 teaspoon of low carb sweetener

- 2 teaspoons of lemon juice

- 2 teaspoons of lime juice

- ½ cup of vegan cream cheese

Mix all ingredients in a small mixing dish and pour into silicone molds or an ice cube tray. Freeze for two hours and serve. Makes enough for 4-5 servings.

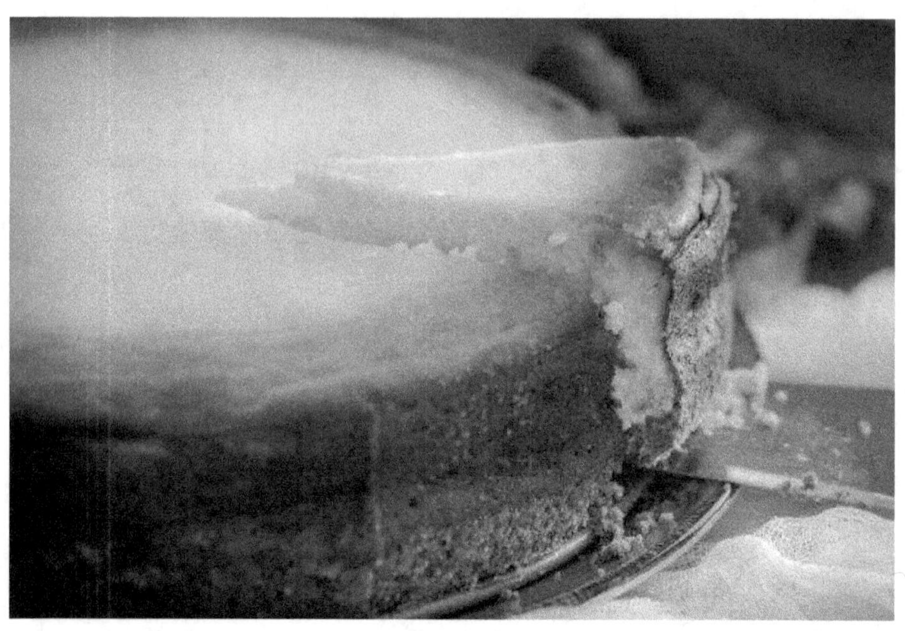

Macaroons

These treats are an ideal blend of coconut and cocoa or dark chocolate. Only a few ingredients are needed to make these no-bake macaroons.

- 1/3 cup of coconut oil

- 1 cup of shredded coconut

- 5 tablespoons of cocoa powder

- 1 teaspoon of vanilla or almond extract

- 3 cups of raw oats

- 2 tablespoons maple syrup

- ½ cups of coconut milk

Combine the coconut milk, oil, vanilla or almond extract, and maple syrup into a bowl and stir together. In a different container, combine the cocoa powder, shredded coconut, and raw oats. Combine both bowls of ingredients and form into balls. Refrigerate for at least two hours before servings.

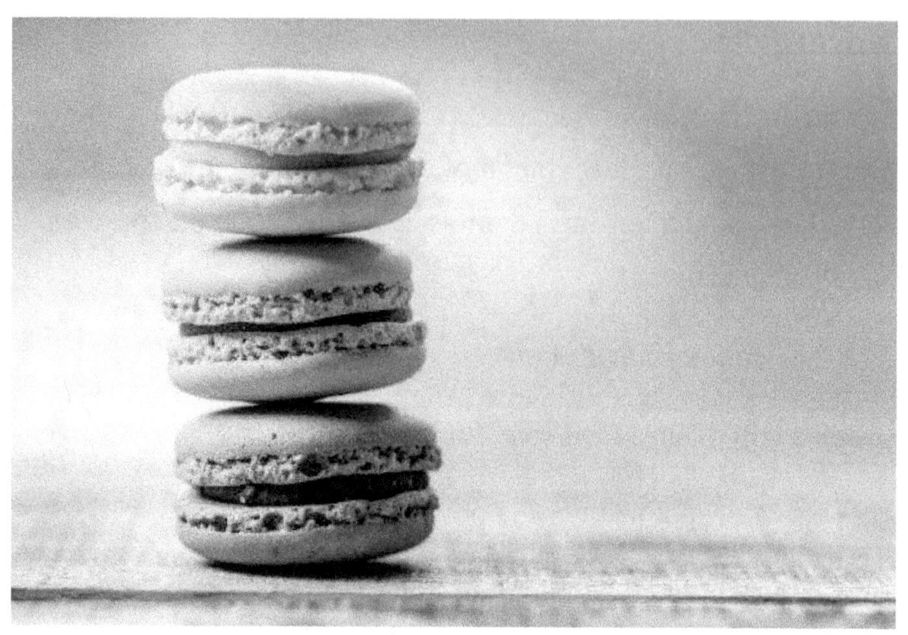

Easy Plant-Based Snacks

Kale Chips

Kale chips are often expensive in specialty grocery and natural food stores, though they are budget-friendly and healthier to make at home. They can be prepared in less than 15 minutes and baked in only 10 minutes, which makes them a quick and easy snack to make. Only three ingredients are needed:

- 2 tablespoons of olive oil

- 1 tablespoon of sea salt

- 1 bunch of kale

Wash and drain one bunch of kale, then remove stems and slice into one or two-inch pieces (chip or bite-sized). Lightly coat each kale piece in olive oil, and place on a large, lined baking sheet. Sprinkle each kale slice with sea salt and preheat the oven, setting to 350 degrees. Bake for 8-10 minutes or until crispy, but not burnt.

Spicy Kale Chips

This recipe involves using one of two spices to create a strong but tasty version of baked kale chips:

- 2 tablespoons of olive oil

- Dash of salt

- 1 teaspoon of cayenne pepper

- 1 teaspoon of chili powder

- 1 bunch of kale

Mix the salt, chili powder, and cayenne powder together, and set aside. Prepare the kale as the recipe above. Use olive oil in coating the kale lightly. Sprinkle a mixture of pepper and salt. Bake for 8-10 minutes and serve. There is the option to skip salt completely and simply use cayenne and/or the chili pepper options.

"Cheesy" Kale Chips

If you enjoy vegan parmesan "cheese", this version of kale chips can be a fun option to try making.

- ½ teaspoons of sea salt

- 2 tablespoons of olive oil

- 1 bunch of kale

- 2 tablespoons of vegan parmesan "cheese"

Prepare the kale like the previous recipes and coat with the olive oil. Place the kale slices on the lined baking tray, and sprinkle salt, then coat with parmesan. Bake for slightly longer, 10-11 minutes, until slightly brown or gold, then remove from the oven and serve.

Roasted Chickpeas

Chickpeas are a great snack to enjoy raw, cooked, or baked into a crispy chip. This recipe provides an easy way to create roasted chickpeas with minimal ingredients.

- ½ of a can of chickpeas

- ½ teaspoon of chili powder (optional)

- 1 teaspoon of salt

- 2 tablespoons of olive oil

Drain and rinse the chickpeas and dry, then pour into a bowl. Lightly coat all chickpeas in olive oil, then mix the chili powder and sea salt together, and coat the beans. Transfer the chickpeas to a lined baking tray and bake for 20-25 minutes on 350 degrees.

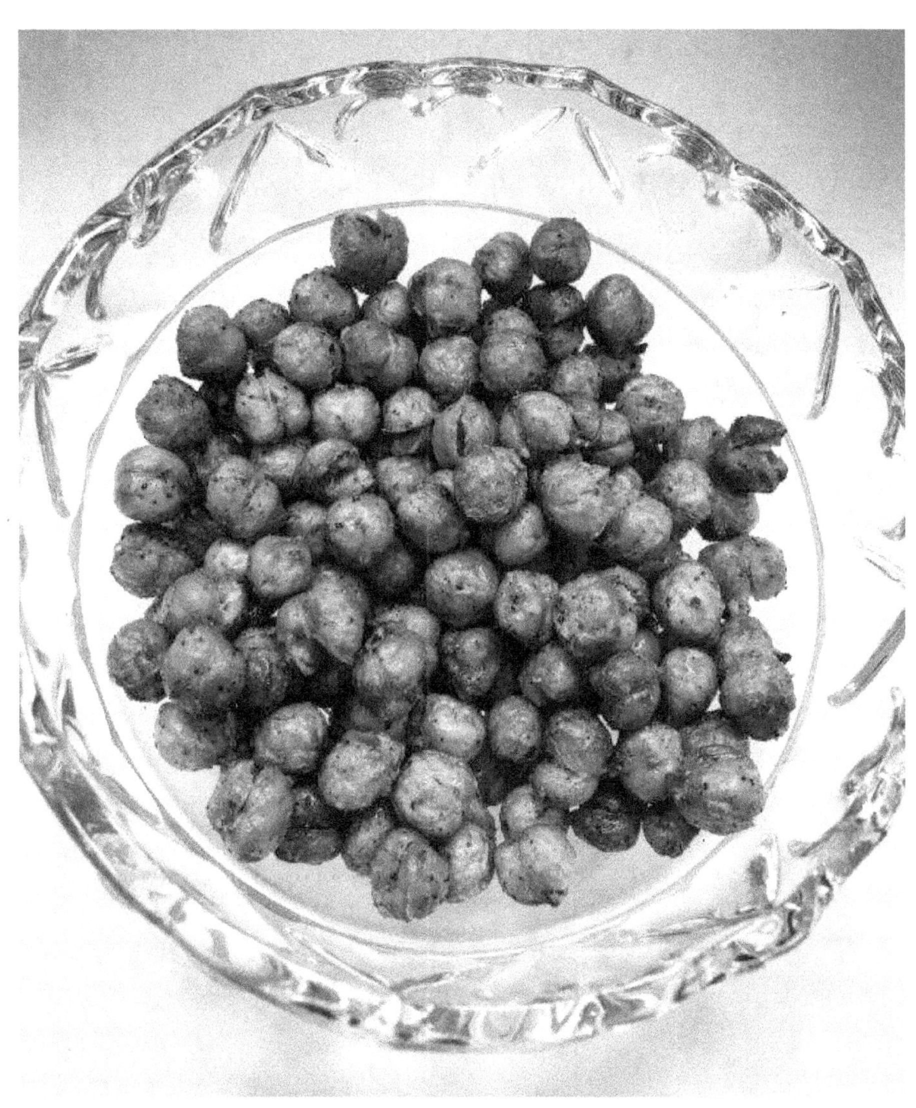

Cinnamon Roasted Pumpkin Seeds

Don't throw away the pumpkin seeds after using a pumpkin for carving or another recipe. The seeds offer a great snack opportunity. Most roasted pumpkin seeds are prepared with salt, though this treat combines cinnamon, instead, for a sweet and savory treat.

- 1 cup of raw pumpkin seeds

- 2 teaspoons of cinnamon

- 2 teaspoons of coconut oil or olive oil

Coat all the pumpkin seeds in olive or coconut oil and arrange on a large baking tray. Sprinkle evenly with cinnamon and bake for 20-25 minutes until slightly crispy, but not burnt.

Chapter 7: 10 Dessert Recipes

Puddings and Yogurt-based Desserts

Vegan or non-dairy yogurt and puddings are delicious options for dessert in plant-based eating. The following recipes are light and tasty, without the guilt of high fats and sugars or dairy products.

Rice Pudding

This recipe uses coconut milk as a creamy foundation for a rich dessert and avoids dairy completely. Basmati rice is used for its nutty, aromatic flavor, and how it blends well with the other ingredients in this recipe.

- 1 cup of basmati rice (uncooked)

- 4 cans of coconut milk (unsweetened) or 6 measured cups

- 1 ½ cups of low carb sweetener (monk fruit or swerve is recommended)

- 1 teaspoon of vanilla extract

- 1 cup of water

- 2 tablespoons of coconut oil or butter

- Cinnamon for the topping

In a large cooking pot, combine the coconut milk, basmati rice, sweetener, and water, and bring to a boil, then reduce heat and continue to cook and simmer for about one hour. Add in the vanilla extract and simmer, stirring regularly until the mixture thickens. Add in the coconut butter or oil and simmer a few more minutes, then remove from heat to cool. Serve sprinkled with cinnamon.

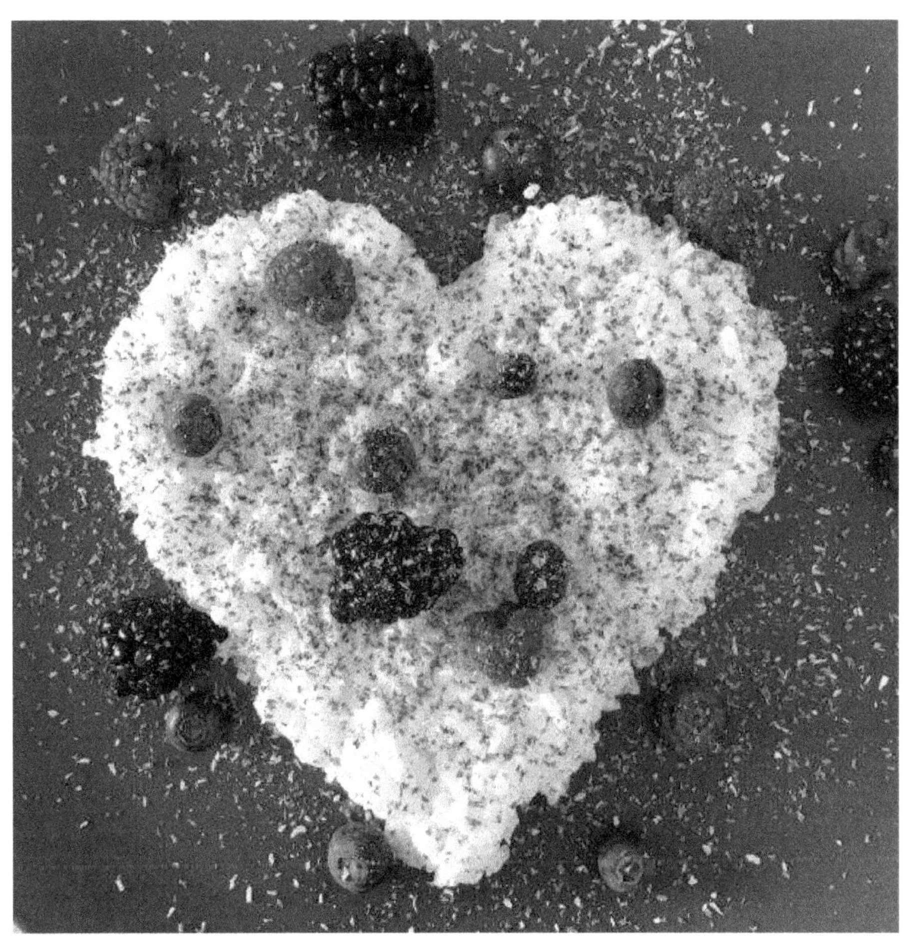

Chia Seed Pudding

If you want a dessert that's healthy and as a meal at the same time, chia seed pudding is the solution. This recipe involves mixing chia seeds with coconut milk, cream, and a variety of toppings for a fun treat, which also provides essential vitamins, protein, and fiber. When chia seeds are soaked in milk or liquid, they become soft and custard-like, which makes them ideal for creating puddings and parfaits.

- 1 cup of chia seeds

- 2 cup of coconut milk

- 2 teaspoons coconut cream or butter

- 1 teaspoon of vanilla extract

- ¼ cup of sweetener (low carb sweetener or maple syrup)

In a small container or bowl, whisk together all the above ingredients. Chia seeds tend to stick to utensils, and it may take a few minutes to thoroughly blends everything. Store in the refrigerator for two hours or more, then remove to serve. The pudding should have a thick, custard-like consistency that is easy to scoop and serve. This recipe serves 2-3 and takes only a few minutes to prepare, before chilling in the refrigerator.

Note: Refrigerating the chia seed pudding overnight allows for the option of enjoying this dessert as breakfast the next morning.

Topping options for this treatment include:

- Cocoa powder or chocolate chips (dark chocolate is recommended)

- Cardamom powder

- Crushed nuts, such as peanuts, pistachios, slivered almonds, crushed pecans, etc.

- Fresh fruits sliced: berries, bananas, melon, peaches, mangos, pineapples, etc.

- Shredded coconut

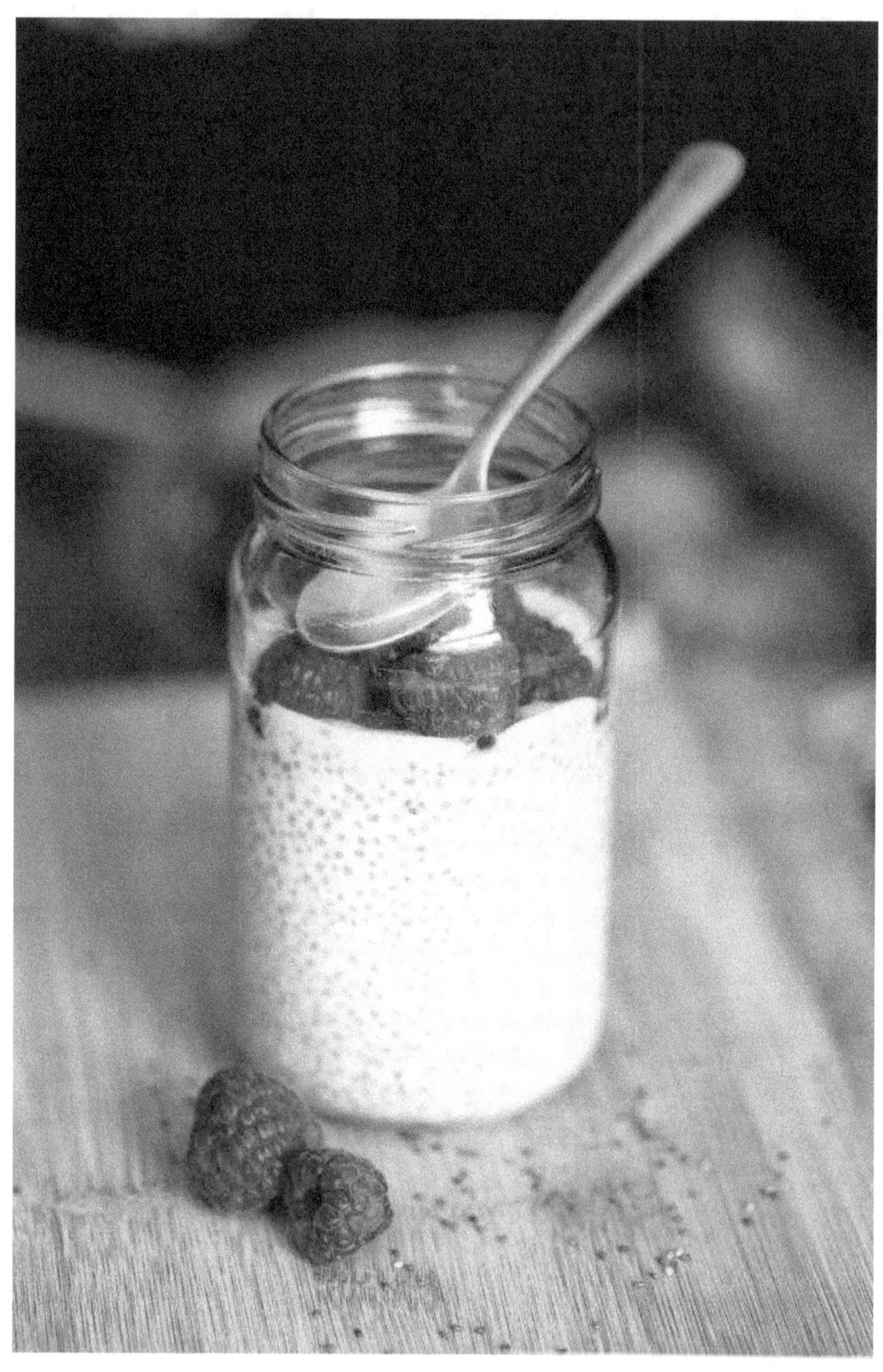

Coconut Yogurt Parfait

The vegan yogurt included in this recipe is made of cultured coconut and can be used in the exact same way as regular, dairy yogurt for this treat.

- ½ cup of crushed peanuts

- 1 cup of sliced berries

- 2 cups of coconut yogurt

- 2 tablespoons of maple syrup

- 2 tablespoons of chocolate chips

- ½ cup of raw oats

In a large sundae glass, add the sliced fruits at the bottom, then scoop heaving spoonful amounts of the coconut yogurt on top and mixing in some of the chocolate chips and maple syrup. On the top layer, top with crushed peanuts oats.

Chia seeds, hemp seeds, and flax can be added to this dish to add more nutrients and protein.

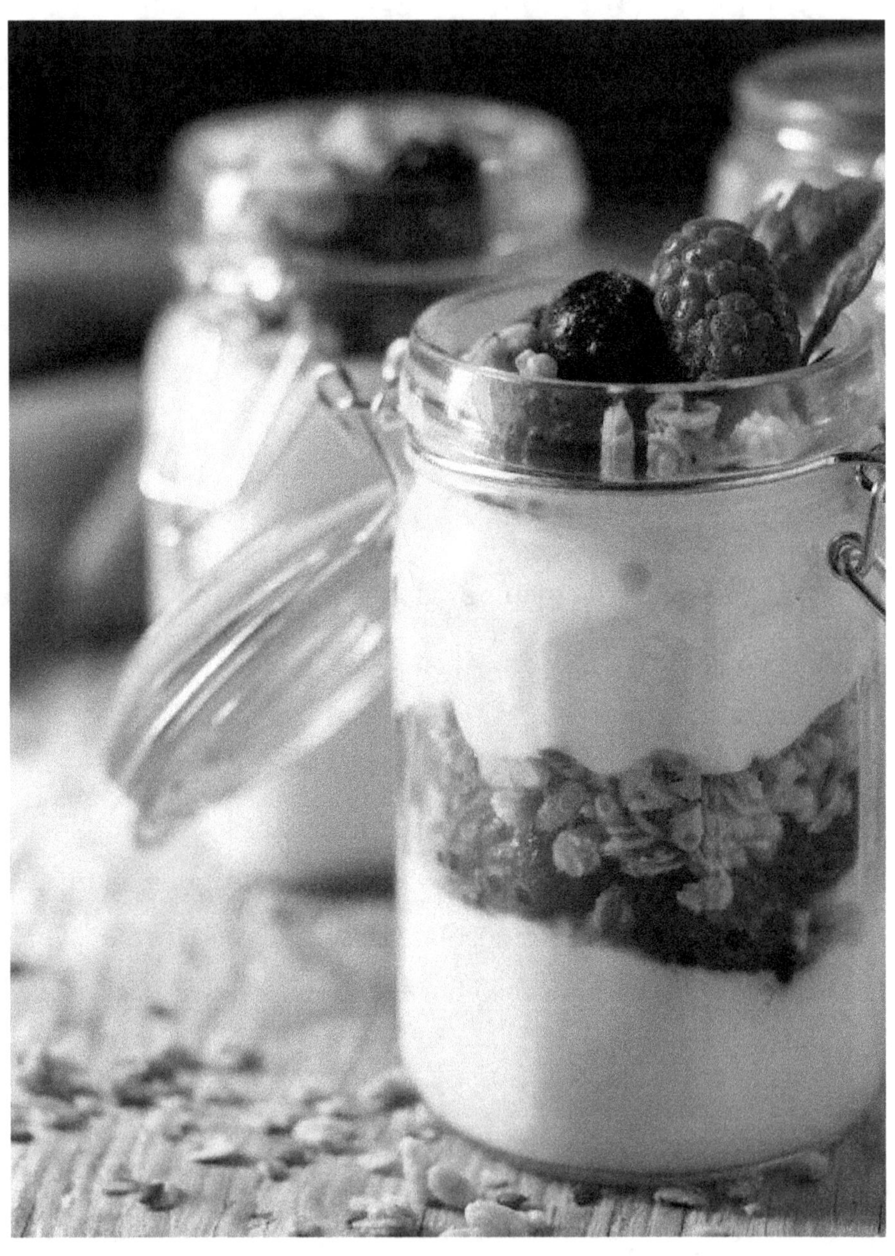

<u>Sticky Rice and Mango Dessert</u>

This dish involves cooking sticky rice with coconut and layering a baking pan, then topped with fresh mango. This dessert is light and refreshing and a good way to finish a meal.

- 2 sliced mangoes (pits removed, sliced)

- 2 cups of sticky rice (uncooked)

- 2 tablespoons of low carb sweetener or maple syrup

- 1 cup of water

- 3 cups of coconut milk

- 1 teaspoon of sesame seeds

Add the water and coconut milk to a cooking pot and bring to a bowl on medium heat. Add in the rice and cook until tender and "sticky". Remove from heat and pour into a large or medium-sized baking dish, making sure the rice evenly coats the bottom of the pan. Cool for 20-25 minutes, then layer the sliced mangoes over the rice, ensuring they cover the entire surface (add more mango if needed). Sprinkle the sesame seeds over the mangoes and serve. If mangoes are not available, peaches make a great substitute.

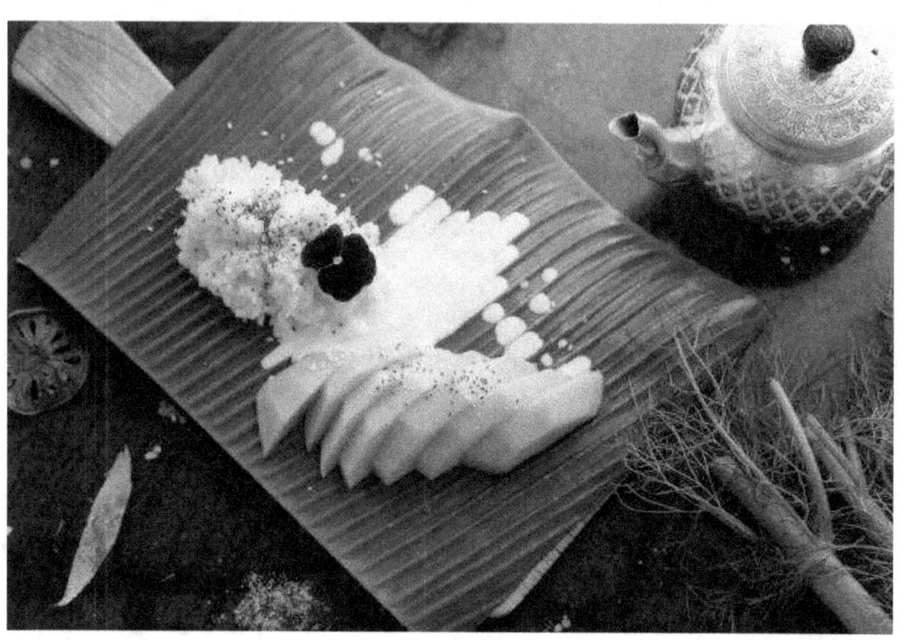

Sweet Potato and Pumpkin Pudding

A sweet and tasty treat, sweet potato pudding can also satisfy an appetite like a main dish and is full of nutrients, such as beta carotene and fiber.

- 1/3 cups of rolled oats

- 1 large cooked sweet potato or yam (baked)

- 1 tablespoon of maple syrup

- 1 teaspoon of cinnamon

- 2 tablespoons of pumpkin puree

- ½ cup of soy or almond milk

Mix the entire ingredients listed above in a blender until it has a smooth consistency. Serves 2-3 and takes only 10 minutes to prepare (not including baking the yam, which can take up to one hour).

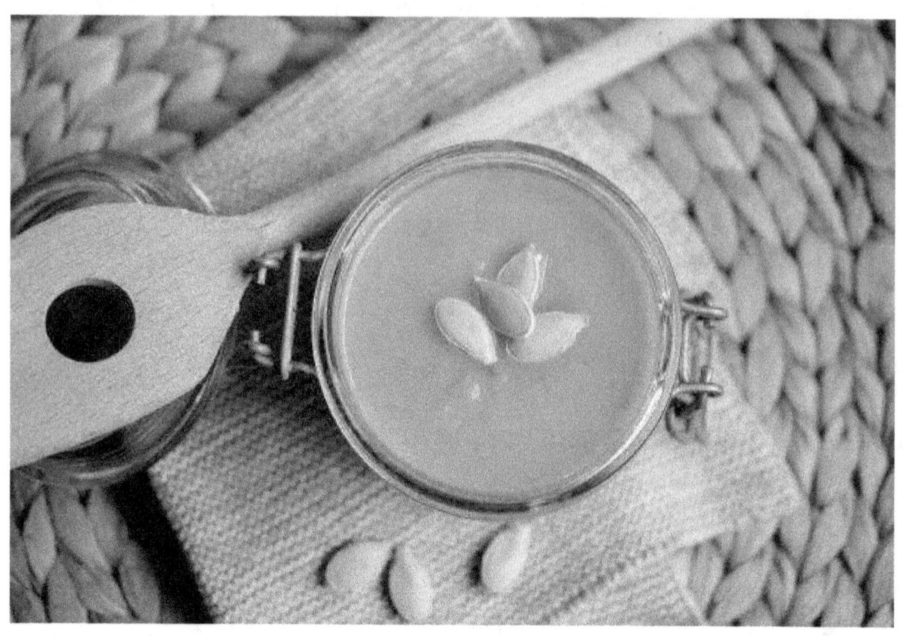

Sweet and Sour Rhubarb Yoghurt Parfait

This recipe is like the regular coconut yogurt parfait, with the addition of stewed rhubarb, which provides a sweet and sour flavor combination.

- 1 cup of blueberries

- 1 cup of stewed rhubarb

- 2 cups of coconut yogurt

- 2 teaspoons of maple syrup

- ½ cups of chia seeds

- ¼ cups of rolled oats

To prepare the rhubarb, slice 2-3 stalks into one-inch pieces before adding in a casserole full of water. Let it start boiling before adding in 2 teaspoons of maple syrup, then reduce in heat and continue to cook on medium until the rhubarb is soft. Remove, drain, and rinse, then place in a bowl to be chilled for almost half an hour.

In a large dessert cup or sundae glass, scoop the rhubarb to the bottom of the cup, then top with several scoops of coconut yogurt, swirling in the maple syrup, then top with the chia seeds, blueberries, and rolled oats. For best results, soak the chia seeds in coconut milk or yogurt of two hours before adding to this recipe.

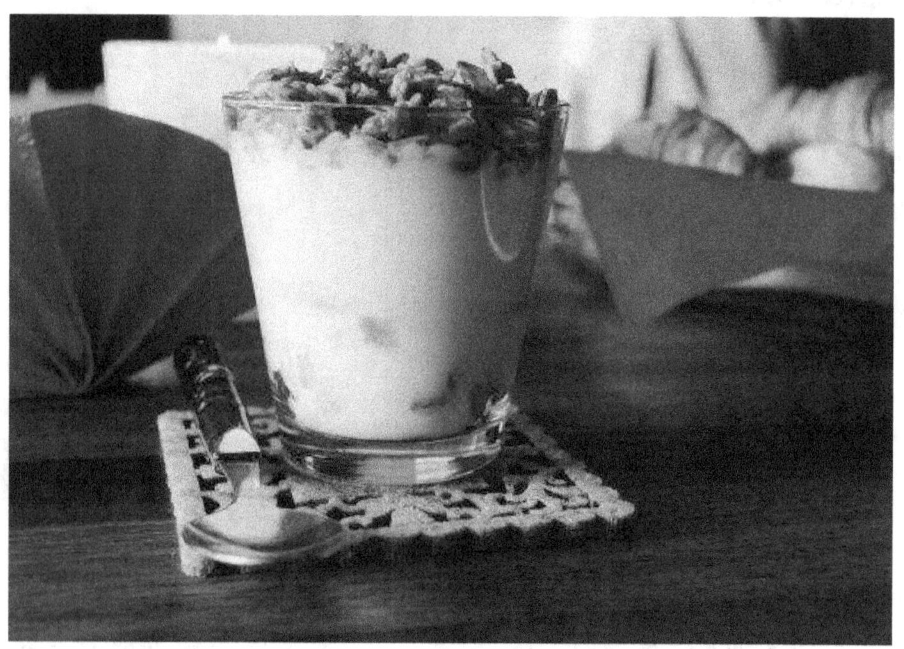

Cakes

Brownie Cake

This vegan chocolate cake resembles a large decadent brownie with a rich texture. It's the ultimate comfort food and made with all plant-based ingredients.

- 1 cup of low carb sweetener (monk fruit or swerve)

- 1 tablespoon coconut flour

- 2 cups of almond flour

- Dash of sea salt

- 1 cup of cocoa powder of baker's chocolate

- ½ cup of coconut oil

- 1 cup of water

- 1 teaspoon of baking powder

- 1 teaspoon of vanilla extract

Mix all the dry ingredients in a large bowl and set aside. Prepare the oven by setting it to 350 degrees. Pour the following items into the bowl with the cocoa, flours, and sweetener: water, coconut oil, and vanilla extract. Blend thoroughly, then pour into a lined or greased baking pan, and bake for 25-30 minutes.

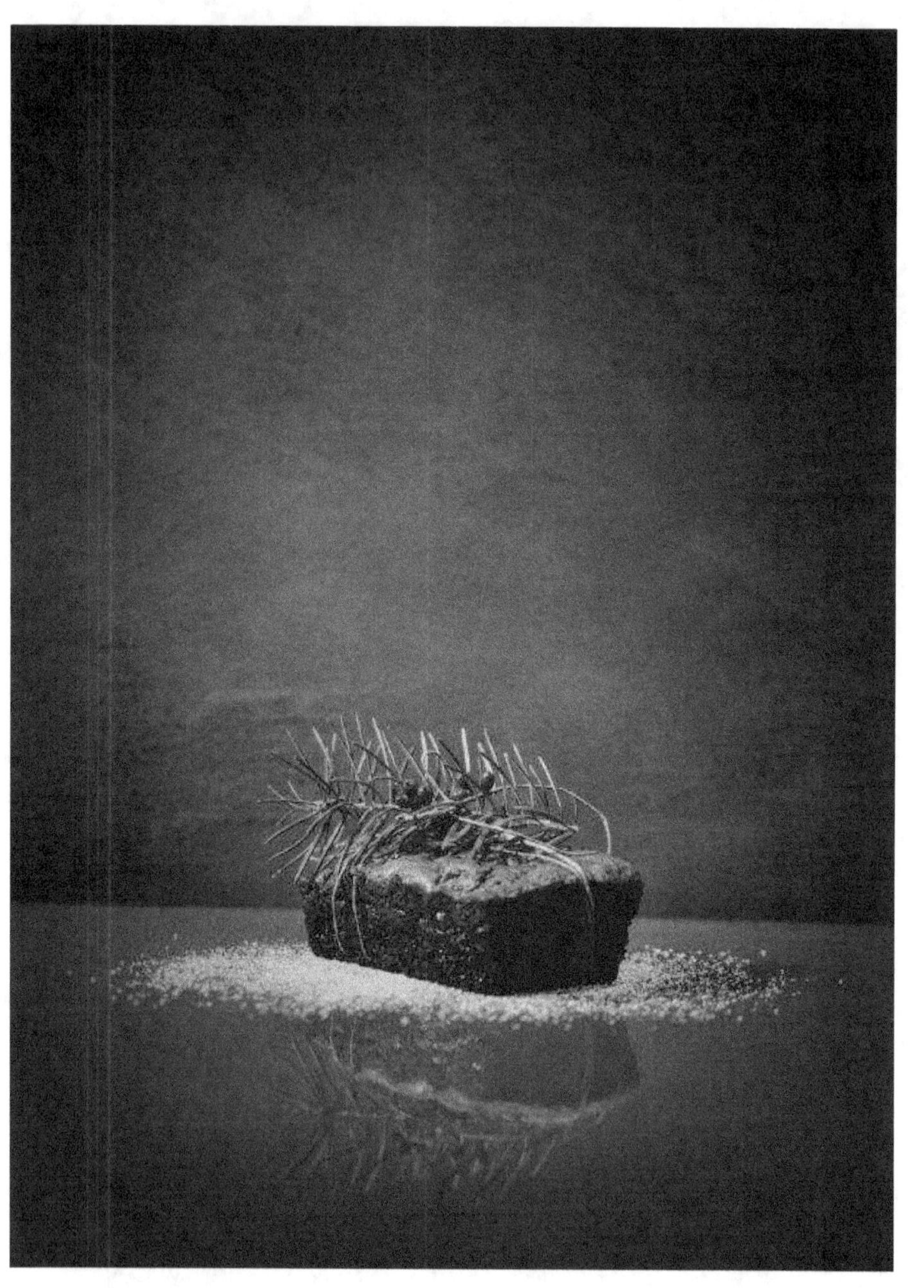

Vanilla Cake

This is a basic cake recipe that can provide a platform for many toppings, syrups, and fruit options. To prepare this cake, combine the dry and wet ingredients in separate bowls, then mix together to bake:

- 1 teaspoon of vanilla extract

- 1 tablespoon apple cider vinegar

- 1 ½ cups of coconut or almond milk

- ½ cup of applesauce (unsweetened)

Combine the above ingredients into a medium bowl, then set aside. Prepare the oven by preheating to 350 degrees. Mix the following ingredient separately in a medium bowl:

- 3 cups of almond flour

- 1 cup of potato starch

- 1 cup of low carb sweetener (monk fruit or swerve)

- 1 teaspoon of baking powder

- 1 teaspoon of baking soda

- Dash of sea salt

- ½ cup of cornstarch

Mix both sets of ingredients together in the larger bowl and prepare a lined cake tin for the oven. Place on a dish ideal for baking before cooking in the oven for about a quarter of an hour or until lightly brown or golden on top. Chill for 10-15 minutes, then serve.

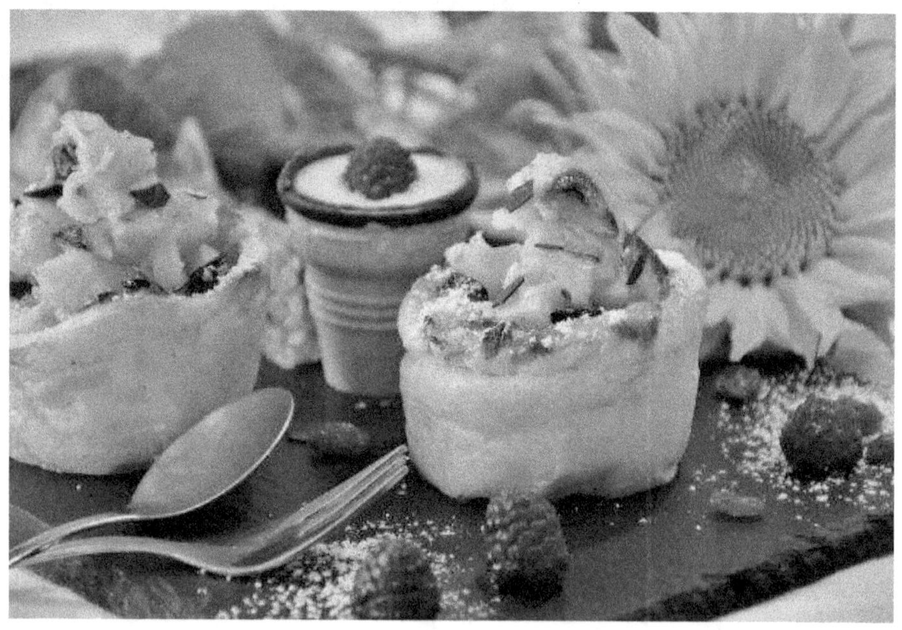

Chapter 8: Starting Your Weight Loss Program: A Four-Week Plan

Weekly Plans and Meals for Each Day of the Week, for Four Weeks

If you're new to a plant-based diet, this four-week plan will give you the tools to start on the right track. During the next four weeks, following these meal plans can help you incorporate a new series of recipes, as well as easy plant-based eating, into an easy-to-follow plan that can set a good foundation for future choices. Getting acquainted with healthy, plant-based foods means incorporating them into your everyday life, so they can be of benefit to you on a regular basis. These plans are also excellent for planning your shopping trips and making choices about the fruits, vegetables, nuts, seeds, soy products, and other foods you select.

Week 1: Plant-based Diet Plan

During your first week, try lots of new and different recipes, or try just a few. Smoothies for breakfast offer a fast and nutritious way to get what you need quickly so that you can move into your day without having to clean up much. Many of the lunch and dinner options are easy to prepare and can be made the night before to make the planning easier. Consider the possibility of leftovers from the lunch or dinner yesterday, and use them the following day, or freeze and/or refrigerate for later in the week. Snacks and desserts are added as an option, though they can be changed or skipped completely if desired.

Week 1	Mon	Tues	Wed	Thurs	Fri	Sat	Sun
Breakfast	Kiwi-Banana and Strawberry Smoothie	Chia seed pudding	Avocado Banana Smoothie	Pumpkin Cinnamon Smoothie	Coconut Yogurt Berry Smoothie	Scrambled Tofu with spinach	Chia seed pudding with fresh fruit
Lunch	Kale and Blueberry salad	Butternut squash soup with rye bread	Lentil dal	Leftover tempeh with yogurt	Green pea soup	Spinach, mandarin and walnut salad	Curried chickpeas
Snack	Apple	Sliced avocado	Hummus on toast	Chocolate brownie	Chia seed pudding	Sliced mangos with peanuts	Black olives with celery sticks

Dinner	Baked tofu	Veggie skillet dish	Sweet and sour tempeh	Tofu, roasted squash, and miso soup	Veggie burgers	Quinoa salad	Veggie skillet dish
Dessert	Yogurt parfait with rhubarb and berries	Fruit salad	Slice of brownie cake	An apple	Sweet and sour tempeh	Zucchini with pasta sauce and noodles	Vanilla cake

Week 2: Plant-based Diet Plan

During your second week, you may notice a difference in the way you feel and eat. You may experience more energy and want to explore new foods or continue to use a lot of the recipes during the first week. Choosing new ingredients or switching them (for example, adding different fruits or combinations of fruits to smoothies) is one way to try something new. Enjoying a baked tofu dinner with vegetables may result in leftover tofu that can be added to a salad or soup the next day. Not only will this help add a variety of different flavors to each meal, but it will also save money on how the foods are used and incorporated into your diet.

Week 1	Mon	Tues	Wed	Thurs	Fri	Sat	Sun
Breakfast	Tropical smoothie	Fruit salad and peanut butter energy bites	Scrambled tofu with arugula	Fruit salad with yogurt	Pumpkin and cinnamon smoothie	Coconut yogurt with sliced banana	Chia seed pudding
Lunch	Miso soup with avocado toast	Cup of chili	Arugula and roasted pear salad	Roasted eggplant with hummus on rye	Toasted rye with avocado	Lentil dal	Leftover lentil dal with a dollop of yogurt
Snack	An orange	A handful of roasted almonds	Rice pudding	Banana	A glass of soymilk with cocoa powder	Kale chips	Fresh fruit bowl
Dinner	Green pea soup		Tofu bake with squash	Stir-fried tempeh with vegetables and rice		Curried chickpeas and sautéed	Sweet ad sour tempeh

						onions	
Dessert	Brownie cake	Vanilla cake	Mango and coconut sticky rice dessert	Banana and a slice of vanilla cake	Leftover brownie slice	Fruit salad	Rice pudding

Week 3: Plant-based Diet Plan

By the third week, you'll become more familiar with how to prepare for grocery shopping and which foods to select. Most people tend to favor certain foods and their flavors over others, and while this is normal, it's also a good idea to continue trying new vegetables, fruits, nuts, and seeds to get a better sense of what's available. All too often, people focus on the limitations of a diet rather than the opportunities available, especially when it comes to a plant-based diet. Eliminating meat and animal byproducts doesn't have to be expensive or restrictive if you're open to trying a wide range of foods and meal options.

Week 1	Mon	Tues	Wed	Thurs	Fri	Sat	Sun
Breakfast	Pumpkin Cinnamon	Yogurt with fres	Chia seed pudding	Mango and pistachio	Tofu scramble with	Chia seed pudding with	Sliced apples, spinach, ch,

	smoothie	h fruits		smoothie	sliced apple	chocolate chips	and crush walnuts and peanuts
Lunch	Ginger carrot soup	Veggie skillet meal	Kale blueberry salad	Stir-fried snow peas and slivered almonds	Baked tofu	Spinach salad with roasted pear	Baked tofu with sweet and sour sauce and rice
Snack	Sliced avocado	Kale chips	Spicy kale chips	Roasted chick peas	Banana	Sliced apples and/or pears	Roasted chick peas
Dinner	Miso soup with button mushrooms	Baked tofu with bok choy	Curried coconut with tofu and vegetables		Zucchini pasta dinner	Leftover pasta	Vegan chili
Dessert	Fresh fruit	Vanilla cake		Rice pudding	Rice pudding with pineapple	Brownie cake	

				and shredded coconut	

In the final week, you will likely notice weight loss, even if you didn't expect to! A plant-based diet is low in calories, trans fats, and high in healthy fats, fiber, and protein, all of which keep your weight well-maintained and within a healthy level. At this stage, you may already be set up or planning your next week, using foods from this four-week plan and more. Always opt for new and exciting foods. Check out specialty shops where exotic fruits and vegetables are an option. Make a point of trying at least one new food each week or every two weeks, and you may find your preferences for food, and your palate will expand over time.

Week 1	Mon	Tues	Wed	Thurs	Fri	Sat	Sun
Break fast	Banana and berry smoothie	Mango and pistachio smoothie	Chia seed pudding	Cherries and peaches smoothie	Chia seed pudding with sliced pineapple and shredded coconut	Avocado banana smoothie	Tofu scramble

Lunch	Lentil dal with burgers	Green pea soup	Lentil dal	Curried carrot and ginger soup	Veggie burger on a bun	Curried cabbage	Sweet and sour tempeh
Snack	Roasted pumpkin seeds	Roasted chickpeas	Banana	Spicy kale chips	A handful of ripe berries	Sliced avocado	Roasted chickpeas
Dinner	Tofu bake and squash	Tofu bake with quinoa salad	Vegetable wrap with tofu, and fresh vegetables	Avocado toast	Curried chickpeas	Lentil dal	Green pea soup
Dessert	Vanilla cake		Brownie cake		Yogurt with berries	Rice pudding	Chia seed pudding with cinnamon

Chapter 9: Conclusion

The plant-based diet offers a wide variety of options for meal preparation. Whether you're a beginner or more experienced with vegan eating, there are major benefits for weight loss and health overall. Choosing plant-based is an ethical and rewarding way of eating that will help you lose excess weight and maintain it at a healthy level. It's more than a diet, but rather, a long-term goal of eating and living well that can significantly improve your life.

Frequently Asked Questions

Question: Is it more expensive to follow a plant-based diet?

Answer: It depends on the food you choose that determines how expensive a vegan diet is. For example, if you eat a lot of prepared foods, such as pre-made salads and specialty foods, such as flavored tofu and/or other items that are outside of the regular whole foods, the price can increase significantly. Unfortunately, fresh produce can be expensive in some regions where it must be shipped and there are limited options, though in general, eating vegan should not cost a fortune. Reviewing the basic foods included in a plant-based diet and selecting the least expensive can help:

- Beans, legumes, and grains can be purchased in bulk or inconvenient cans at a decent price.

- Fresh vegetables and fruits can be expensive, though choosing a frozen option may be more convenient and less costly.

- Since meat and dairy are avoided, and these foods can add up to cost a lot, the only additional expense on your grocery bill are soy-based and other vegan foods that replace meat and dairy. The cost can range, though often, there are less expensive options available that make it easy for everyone.

- Nuts and seeds can be pricy for anyone, though buying in bulk is one way to focus on only the amounts you need while keeping within a budget.

Question: Is the vegan diet good for athletes?

Answer: Absolutely! In fact, you'll likely get more protein, calcium, and nutrients in general on a vegan diet. Choosing dark leafy green vegetables provides a wealth of vitamins, fiber, and protein that a lot of meat doesn't contain, and your body will metabolize and process plant-based foods easier, making weight loss success and getting into good shape a goal that can be achieved with the right commitment. There are a growing number of famous athletes and celebrities who adhere to a vegan diet with excellent results.

Question: How do I know if some of the foods I buy or choose are animal-free?

Answer: Choosing fresh fruits and vegetables is a surefire way to avoiding any meat products, as well as any other foods that are purchased in their whole form, including nuts, seeds, herbs, and spices. Tofu is soybean-based and almost never contains any meat or animal byproducts. To be certain, read all labels on the food items you buy, as many will have a label or sticker that notes if they are vegan, gluten-free, and/or nut-free. These labels are especially helpful for people who have allergies and need to avoid certain types of foods and ingredients.

Question: Are there any dangers of going vegan, such as vitamin or nutrient deficiencies or other conditions?

Answer: Fortunately, all your required nutrients can be easily consumed and included in a plant-based diet. This includes B12 and vitamin D. Vitamin B12 is found in fermented soy, such as miso and tempeh, as well as brewer's yeast. Vitamin D is absorbed through our skin from the sun, though it is also available in fortified milk and non-dairy milk beverages. Adequate amounts of protein, calcium, iron, and all other nutrient requirements are found in a wide range of plant-based foods. At one time, many people avoided eating vegan out of fear they would lose nutrients, which is quite the opposite. In fact, you'll find you're getting more out of a vegan or plant-based diet than if you choose meat and dairy.

Question: Should I switch my body care products, such as soaps, shampoos, moisturizers, and other items to vegan and cruelty-free options?

Answer: As a part of the vegan lifestyle, this is an excellent option, and there are a growing number of retailers who promote and design cruelty-free makeup, lotions, skincare, and body care products. This can extend to many other products, including lines of clothing and materials used in making a variety of items, including furniture. While some of these product lines can be expensive, some people who want a completely animal-free life can opt to choose these options as well. You may find that some vegan products, especially for body and skin, may be easier on your body and with less irritation or negative effects. As with any type of product, it's best to try them first, to determine if its right for you and your life, before continuing to use it.

Question: If I'm gluten intolerant or have Celiac disease, can I follow a vegan diet?

Answer: Yes, and it might actually be better for you, as you'll have a lot of plant-based options that are naturally gluten and wheat-free. As with any diet, you'll simply need to avoid the same products, such as whole wheat, bread, and baking products and other snacks or sauces that contain gluten or gluten-related products.

Question: Can I follow a plant-based diet if I have a lot of allergies?

Answer: Yes, and it's easier than you think. Because most foods are not processed, there is a benefit to eating whole, natural foods in place of packaged options. This may, in time, alleviate allergies in some people. If your allergy is specific to an additive or ingredient that is found in packaged food, it will most likely be avoided in a vegan diet. Allergies to certain fruits and vegetables, while possible, can simply entail avoiding them completely, whether it's a citrus fruit or a specific vegetable that you cannot consume.

Question: How can I eat and choose vegan foods at holiday and other family events or social engagements?

Answer: Guaranteed, there are usually vegan options available. If you have the option to find out in advance, arrange so that your preference for plant-based foods is an option. For more informal family gatherings, bring a plate or two of your own vegan creations, and you may be pleasantly surprised by how well-received it is. Many people who have never tried a vegan diet do not realize how many options there are for meal planning and taste. If you've lost any weight or appear healthier and leaner, people will take notice and attribute this to your vegan diet, which makes a significant impact.

Question: Do vegans live longer, and can we live longer without disease as the result of a plant-based diet?

Answer: There are some promising studies that claim vegans may outlive their meat-eating counterparts. There is also research that may indicate lower incidents of disease, including cancer, heart disease, and memory loss conditions often associated with aging and other dietary factors. Eliminating animal fats and products from your diet can cause you to feel more energetic as well, which can motivate you to keep active and lose weight if needed, or tone and gain a better fitness level overall.

Question: How do I get the most out of vegan eating? Is it more variety or should I focus on the nutrition levels instead?

Answer: A variety of foods is going to keep people interested in plant-based eating, though adding foods and balancing your dietary choices based on nutrient content and levels are also vital to a healthy and balanced lifestyle. When considering which foods are best for protein, calcium, fiber, and antioxidants, consider dark leafy greens as a top choice for covering all these nutrients. Choose "superfoods" as much as possible, such as chia seeds, avocado, and coconut. If you want to increase the nutrient power in your smoothies, add flax or hemp protein powder or crushed seeds to your drink before processing in the blender. This will ensure you get more than enough in just one serving.

Question: Is vegan safe for people of advanced age? Our kids also allowed to follow a plant-based diet? Are there any age limitations?

Answer: In short, no, there shouldn't be any limitations, as plant-based eating is safe for everyone of all dietary needs. Providing a vegan diet for kids is a healthy option, though it's best to check with a physician, just in case they require additional nutrients and/or supplements. This may be especially crucial for kids with chronic health conditions or may need certain types of nutrients more than others. For mature adults, the same applies. Check with your doctor first, then determine how to get any additional supplements and vitamins you might need. In general, the vegan diet is healthy and shouldn't cause any negative reaction, unless you're avoiding a lot of nutrients and narrowing down your own selection.

Question: How can I work around a soy allergy on a vegan diet?

Answer: Soy-based foods make up a significant part of the vegan diet, though they can be replaced with other protein-based alternatives, such as nut-based kinds of milk, seitan, and choosing vegetables high in iron, protein, and calcium. Now more than ever, there are plenty of options for vegans, including both soy and non-soy products.

Question: How successful is long-term weight loss on a plant-based diet?

Answer: It's successful because your body is consuming less fat, carbohydrates, and unnatural foods overall, making it easier to lose weight, digest, and metabolize better, and keep the weight off.

Question: How can I introduce other people to a vegan diet? Are there any suggestions?

Answer: Focus on the choices that a plant-based or vegan diet provides, instead of the restrictions (no meat, no dairy, etc.). Anyone new to a plant-based diet may be pleasantly surprised by how many options are available to them and how much more accommodating stores, restaurants, and markets are towards the vegan lifestyle. It is also a lifestyle about compassion and mindfulness, which takes into consideration all the foods chosen for their quality and animal-free status. Motivating people to start a vegan diet can be challenging because the first (and key) item most will ask is: What do I eat without meat? How can I have dairy and cheese on a vegan diet? Going vegan should be done gradually, over time, for some people who are resistant to change, but want to adapt to it over time.

Question: Is it easier to eliminate meat-based and dairy foods in stages, or jump into the vegan diet completely at once?

Answer: For most people, starting with small changes is ideal, and gradually losing and replacing animal products and foods with plant-based options is usually recommended. There are some people who are eager to "jump" into the vegan way of life, and they may naturally be good at adapting, or simply want to reap the awards sooner rather than later. This may cause some people to switch back to non-vegan eating if they don't prepare ahead, as they may become discouraged at some point. If you jump into a plant-based diet, be prepared for your body to react to the sudden changes, but also note that once you become adjusted, the rewards will definitely be worthwhile.

Question: When I choose a restaurant, how likely the staff to accommodate a vegan diet?

Answer: Most restaurants offer vegan foods and are exceptional at accommodating their customers. It's always best to check in advance just to be certain. When in doubt, always have a few vegan snacks handy, just in case there is a lack of plant-based food, though often, you'll be pleasantly surprised at how most places will offer vegan food options.

Description

How can a plant-based diet enable you to lose the excess weight you need and improve your health? Eating well and trying new recipes is a great way to motivate weight loss. One of the healthiest and most sustainable ways to eat well is by following a plant-based or vegan diet. In this book, you'll discover 50 delicious recipes, all of which are easy to prepare and are made from common ingredients you are already aware of. Contrary to many opinions, a vegan diet doesn't have to be expensive or considered a specialized diet, when there are limitless varieties of fruits, vegetables, grains, nuts, seeds, and many other non-dairy and meat-free options.

This book will provide a wide range of information and recipes to start you on a successful path to plant-based eating, including:

- The importance of plant-based eating for your body and health

- How adapting to a vegan diet is easier on your digestive system and weight loss

- The impact of eating processed foods and meat on weight gain and disease

- Focusing on simple, easy-to-make recipes that don't cost a fortune and can be made with just a handful of ingredients

- Getting rid of bad eating habits and replacing them with new, healthier practices.

- Choosing the best foods for your diet: keeping it healthy and vegan

- Focusing on plant-based proteins and nutrients

When you begin a new plant-based diet, you'll need a variety of tasty recipes to begin:

- Breakfast smoothies with all-natural ingredients

- Soups and salads that can be enjoyed as meals or side dishes

- Main dinner recipes easy to make

- Snacks and desserts

Starting a plant-based diet doesn't have to be difficult or challenging if you have the right foods and recipes to choose from. A vegan diet opens a new world of taste that isn't often discovered in a meat-based diet. There are also many ways to enjoy some of the most common fruits and vegetables in our local grocery stores, as well as exploring many other plant-based foods that are both convenient and delicious. Overall, the goal of a plant-based diet is to achieve optimum health and achieve a healthy weight, both of which become much more attainable with veganism. Losing weight is part of the process while gaining a better level of health and living ethically are also major advantages of the diet. Once you discover the limitless options there are in plant-based eating, it will only become more enjoyable and adventurous when it comes to exploring a wide range of foods. This book is your first step to reaching your goal of weight loss and a better way of eating, not just in the short-term, but as part of a lifestyle that will improve the quality of your overall well-being.

www.ingramcontent.com/pod-product-compliance
Lightning Source LLC
Chambersburg PA
CBHW070707250726
48662CB00001B/291